Middle Age Madness

My Menopause Diary

By
Sarah Stenton

Contents

Dedication

To all the fabulous people who follow my page, thank you for making this possible.

And to David, Holly & Ella: Love you, thank you for all the encouragement and sorry for writing about sex!

Acknowledgments

To my fabulous friends, Julie, Jo, Valerie & Caroline - unwittingly background characters to a lot of the drama in this book – is it gin o'clock?

To my mum, dad and sister, Jo, who, despite quite possibly burning with shame, have followed my blog from the start and keep cheering me on – love you.

To all my family and friends, and anybody who knows me, thank you for not mentioning my hairy Mary every time we meet.

And to all the women suffering with the menopause – you are not alone.

About the Author

Sarah was born in Oxford, has lived in Manchester and South West France, and now lives in Shropshire with her husband, two daughters, and two dogs. She started her popular Facebook blog, Middle Age Madness, in 2018, and is especially proud that men, as well and women, find it relatable and funny.

Introduction

This is a book about the struggles and outrage of the menopause. It all started with one poem that I posted on Facebook and led to me writing a diary, expressing my bemusement at what was happening to my body and my mind. In order to survive the menopause, it is my firm belief that a sense of humour is a must, along with an extensive vocabulary of rather fine swear words.

How It All Began

Sweaty boobs, back fat

Melting flaps and all of that

Leaky ladies, a bristly chin

We middle age girls cannot win

Drying up, inside and out

Hairy toes and hairy snout

Knickers pulled up nice and high

Boobs somewhere around your thigh

Can't even sneeze without a piddle

Nice roll of fat around our middle

But we are made of stronger stuff

Though we may have a saggy muff

We will age with charm and grace

And hair removal cream on our face

We will laugh instead of cry

As the years go flying by

We are kind and strong and proud

And, after a few gins, very loud

Anti-wrinkle cream will do its best

But vodka and laughter can do the rest

So, age, my friends, with a smile on your face

And a Tena lady firmly in place

Dear Diary

January 21st 2018

Today I'm going to talk about Sarah. Sarah is a middle aged woman going through the menopause. Sarah fucking hates the menopause. It makes her feel fat. It has made her grow a beard. It makes her tired yet gives her insomnia. Sarah has mood swings that are unfathomable even to her and must be bewildering to others. Sarah tries to keep her emotions contained but this makes her want to cry with rage and self pity that nobody notices how marvellous she is being by not roaring/crying/laughing uncontrollably.

Sarah is outraged that she can't go round calling people a twat, arse, shit head or knob jockey. It would make her feel better. When Sarah is prime minister she will pass a law allowing menopausal women to say what the fuck they like. It will be cheaper than HRT and more beneficial.

Sometimes Sarah feels invisible and as sexy as last nights leftovers.

Sarah tries hard to make herself look nice. Sarah plucks her chin every fecking morning, puts her make up on, wears something nice yet still feels like a sack of shite most of the time.

Sarah knows these low moments are the menopause playing havoc with her hormones and emotions. Sarah really wants the menopause to shag off with bells on at times like this.

Sometimes Sarah gets fed up of being Sarah and dreams of running away like Shirley Valentine. Then she remembers that she has a lovely husband, two children, fabulous friends, and, most importantly, two beautiful dogs that she could never leave, so Shirley goes back in her box. Then Sarah gets pissy about the sofa scatter cushions being placed in the wrong order and googles flights to Greece.

Sarah gets annoyed very easily. Sarah gets upset very easily. Sarah feels as if nobody understands her. Sarah has hairy nipples and overgrown fanny flaps. Sarah has a little wee when she sneezes. Sarah couldn't hold a shit in if you paid her to. No fucking wonder Sarah gets fed up.

Sarah likes Gin. It is balm on her nerves. Sarah thinks she might drink a few hefty Gin's this weekend as she has to tackle her overgrown biff bush in readiness for a spa weekend with her husband. The spa weekend is two weeks away but Sarah knows it will take several attempts and at least 18 razors to get the biff bush tidy. Sarah knows that if she does not carry out this maintenance work people will be caught up in the biff bush and dragged under water. Despite the menopause fucking with her head, Sarah is still thinking of other people.

Sarah is winning. Just about. Christ on a bike it is tough though.

Spikes and Shirley Valentine
31st August 2019

I have been having strange menopausal spikes recently. Very anxious and stressed followed by rage and snarkyness and occasional bouts of terrifying randyness, and of course crying and wailing. My hormones are going haywire at the moment and can be summed up in a car journey we had the other day.

Randy spike - knickers came off in the car (I wasn't driving)

Husband raised an eyebrow and put his foot down.

Anxious spike - What if we have an accident and I'm found with no knickers on? Or worse - what if I sneeze? (knickers back on).

Husband looked a tad despondent.

Snarky spike - It's alright for you I have to live with these fecking hormones in my body!

Emotional spike - My hairy, fat body! sob!

All in the space of 5 minutes.

So, I declined an invitation to go out with husband and last night I had the lesser spotted evening in on my own. I rubbed my hands with glee and poured a large gin and tonic and kissed the glass far more lovingly than I kiss anything else.

I did a quick scan of the house and found that it was a shit tip. No problem, I whizzed round, shoving, stuffing and pushing things, clean or not, into cupboards and under beds, did a dance with the duster and a quick hoover, followed by a bathroom blitz. Now I could sit down and enjoy a film of my choice with a gin, a bag of crisps and a chocolate eclair for dinner. Perfect. On went Shirley Valentine and I drifted off to Greece with our middle-aged heroine.

Just as Shirley and Costas were about to ride on the boat, in every sense of the word, husband came home, earlier than expected, stood in front of the telly and tried to have a conversation with me. At one point I was leaning so far over to the left trying to get round him to see our Shirl that I would've given a contortionist a run for his money. I got stitch in my side. Husband noticed that I was slightly less than interested in talking to him.

'Rude' he said

'Shirley Valentine' I said, the top half of my body still at a right angle with the bottom.

'You've seen this loads, talk to me instead'

'For fecks sake! One night! One night to myself! Not even a night! Just a few hours! That is all I ask!' I ranted; a tad overwrought.

Husband backed away. He knows the signs by now.

Shirley jumped into the sea in the raw. Good girl yourself.

All was well again.

Then our youngest daughter had the audacity to return from her two-week holiday. Husband smirked, knowing I'd have to talk to our child at least for a minute or two. But no! Beloved daughter had lots of news and stories to share with her mother, who by this point had a strange rictus grin stuck on her face and a manic, desperate look in her eyes. I'm not such a shite mother that I can completely ignore my offspring so I went for one word in three and tried to keep my mind off dear Shirley.

By the time the tales had ended the living room was full of husband, dogs, daughter and any hope of watching the rest of Shirley in peace was laughable, frankly. So, I necked my gin, tipped the crisps into my mouth and shoved in the whole chocolate eclair in one go. It wasn't chips and egg but it was very satisfying.

My advice to all the husbands out there - your wife is fabulous but she sometimes needs cocktails, TLC and Shirley Valentine.

Husband's advice to the men? If the knickers come off in the car stop the fecking thing and jump on board.

Re-tuning to Tena Lady
November 5th 2019

Yesterday was the day that all the stars aligned and I finally slid headlong into middle age.

I got in the car yesterday morning and turned on Radio 2. It was just fecking noise.

I remember the glory days of Radio 1 - Mike Read for Breakfast, Simon Bates, Gary Davies with his bit in the middle etc. At some point either I changed or it changed and I tuned into Radio 2 and discovered the glory of Terry Wogan followed by Ken and the joy of pop master. And many happy years I spent with those two in my ear-holes.

However, yesterday my eardrums refused to tolerate the early morning noise and nonsense. Acting almost by its own accord, my hand reached forward and re-tuned the radio to Smooth Extra. Fecking Smooth Extra! Part of me was mortified but oh, the instant bliss! A calming, tranquil mood settled over me and eased my nerves shredded by the recent radio screeching.

I floated through the day on a cloud of easy listening and wafted home, picking up the post as I got in.

Tena lady had sent me a leaflet offering a free pack of coupons for Silhouette piss proof underwear.

I crashed down a little bit from my waftiness and ranted at the cheek of Tena. 'Fuck this! Why are they sending me offers on piss pants? Do they think I am an old lady?'

It was pointed out that I can't leave the house without a Tena lady. Harsh but true.

'Yes. But they don't know that do they? They are assuming that because I am 48, I can't hold in a wee and my pelvic floor is around my knee caps' I huffed and puffed

'I could have the tightest fanny in the UK!' I said, unwisely.

On cue I sneezed, violently. As the inevitable trickle of piss made itself known husband ran to get the mop, nudging the Tena leaflet a little bit closer to me.

He reminded me, through the toilet door, that I get excited by seed catalogues so I can't really rant about receiving targeted middle-aged mail.

I tidied myself up and then went to make dinner, glass of G & T in hand, pelvic floor held in place by way of a fresh flap pad and Smooth Extra gently playing in the background on the wireless.

Rock on!

Accidents Happen

12th March 2020

I've just had one of those phone calls....

'Hello madam', he said, 'I understand you have had an accident that wasn't your fault?'

'Darling, I have an accident every fucking day! You push two melons out of your piss slot in 14 months and try telling me you don't have accidents years down the fucking line'.

The line went dead.

Perhaps not the sort of accident he was referring to but bad luck for phoning after I had just sneezed matey.

Lockdown
Monday 4th May 2020

This is how I spend my days.

7.40 am: Wake up, realise I am still alive, wonder what day it is, stretch, fart, feel a bit of wee escape and try to hurry to the loo.

7.43 am: still trying to get up off my back to go to the loo. Everything is aching.

7.45 am: Still flaying about on the bed like a beetle on its back, trying to get into sitting up position. Roll over onto side, slide stiff legs out of bed and rest of body follows in an elegant, slug like movement.

7.47 am: Finally on loo. Then clean teeth, clean the sink after every fucker has left their spitty toothpaste in it. Look in the mirror. Right arm reaches for the tweezers like a reflex.

8.15 am: Finish plucking beard and tash. Will do nose tomorrow, didn't have a piss pad in place to cope with mad sneezing fit that plucking nasal hair brings.

8.30 am: cleaning fit downstairs, sweeping, hoovering, tidying, followed by removal of one of best cushions from randy Labrador who is trying to hump it.

8.58 am: Rearrange scatter cushions in correct order so my head won't explode, and spray liberally with Febreze. Fecking dog.

9.00 am: Do Joe Wicks. Star jumping bastard.

9.33 am pause Joe to die for 5 minutes and catch breath

9.55 am: Loo again, post Joe Wicks. Inevitable really.

10.05 am: look in mirror, want to see healthy, glowing, energised, hair free face. See sweating, red faced, puffing, gasping half dead person.

10.25 am: Breakfast. Bacon sandwich. It's allowed because I did Joe.

11 am: wonder aimlessly from room to room picking up stuff and putting it back.

11.20 am Bored.

11.22 am: make a coffee and have a biscuit.

11.45 am: Give roll of flab a squidge to see if it has gone down from yesterday. Must stick to diet.

11.47 am: Wonder what to make for lunch.

12.30 pm: excited! Daughter is a key worker (Saturday girl in newsagents but has been doing extra shifts during the week whilst in lockdown) Husband will be bringing her back soon and we can have lunch.

1.30 pm. Lunch and lovely family chat round the table.

2.00 pm: post lunch slump. Kids on phones, husband reading.

2.01 pm: I wonder what to make for tea.

3 pm: to stop self falling into a nana nap coma and drooling on the sofa, husband and I decide to take the dogs for a walk.

3.03 pm: still trying to get out of chair.

3.10 pm: trying to lift leg high enough to get it in welly.

3.20 pm: finally on our way.

4.00 pm: In the middle of lovely walk, husband and I talk about all the things we have missed during lockdown.

'sex' is top of husbands list (difficult to have relations while teenagers are housebound with ears like fecking bats and minds like sewers) 'Friends' is top of my list (actual friends not the TV programme which is on all the fucking time). This is followed, for both of us by family, freedom and the pub. Did we take everything so much for granted before, or is that what we are supposed to do being lucky enough to live in a free country?

5.00 pm Exciting! It is nearly tea time.

5.01 pm Turn on daily briefing.

5.10 pm Turn off daily briefing the minute some twat journalist opens mouth to ask nonsense question. If you know everything and are gifted with hindsight why not go and be in charge yourself? Arse.

5.11 pm. Arrival of daily rage fit. I like this mood swing. Lots of swearing about twat arsed journalists.

5.35 pm arrival of daily anxiety fit. What if I forget to pluck chin hair and come downstairs one morning with chimpanzee chin?

6.30 pm Tea time, exotic fayre from the pantry. Pasta bake using the fucking enormous pillow case size bag of pasta which will last me until death and was the only one I have been able to find.

7.30 pm: post dinner slump. Everyone on phones, or reading, or watching pure solid shite on TV.

9.30 pm: Yawn. announce I am going upstairs to bed.

9.32 pm trying to get out of reclining chair.

9.33 pm: 'thought you were going to bed?' says husband.

9.35 pm still trying to get out of fucking reclining chair. Nearly sobbing with effort and frustration.

9.41 pm: Lie flat on fucking reclining chair, which is incapable of putting itself upright, and slide off in delicate fashion, like shit off a hot shovel.

10 pm: bed and book.

10.01 pm: Can't see book as eyes are old and knackered and reading glasses are other side of the room. Decide to squint.

10.23 pm: feel a sneeze coming on. Get out of bed with all haste and bolt to the loo

10.24 pm: Made it.

10.45 pm. Turn out light and snuggle down to sleep.

10.46 pm: Husband appears, turns on light and gets ready for bed.

11.00 pm: Husband still fucking about folding his clothes, scratching his balls and belching.

11.05 pm: Finally! Husband in bed. Turns out light.

11.06 pm I need a wee.

11.12 pm: Husband snaps at me to stop wriggling. 'Go and have a wee' he says.

11.13 pm Arrival of daily depression and pity fit. 'Why can't I just piss and be done with it? Why do I have to have 23 fecking wee's before I can go to sleep? Why am I fat? Why am I hairy? Why have a I got a fucking beard? Why am I sweating? You don't understand what has happened to me, it's alright for you, just grow a pony tail, buy a motorbike and be done with male menopause, your dick doesn't dry out and your balls don't drop to your knees' etc.

11.30 pm. Wait until husband is in deep sleep, turn on the light and get up for a wee.

2.43 am: Husband waits until my hot flushes have stopped and my insomnia has allowed me to finally go to sleep, turns on light and goes for a wee.

2.48 am: Damn him! now I need a wee.

2.49 am: Mind over matter. I can hold it in.

3.10 am: Dreaming of going to lots of different toilets, all of them like something out of trainspotting, everyone I open has something wrong: filthy, no door, no side, walls made of glass, people walking past. Poor bladder is screaming at me to wake up and go to the loo.

3.14 am: Listen to bladder and visit the loo.

3.18 am. Deep blissful sleep.

7.40 am: peel open eyes and do it all again.

Stay safe and well everyone

Hay there
Wednesday June 4th 2020

My lovely friend Mrs A gave me three bags of hay from her meadow the other day, for my chicken pen.

I dutifully emptied the bags for my girls and used my hands to shove it into the hen house and round the enclosure. It was dry and brittle, having been exposed to a lovely dose of spring sunshine.

My hair got in my eyes and I moved it back. That's strange, I thought, how I have managed to get hay on my head? I shoved it back again. The hay was still there. I looked at my hands to see if I had hay on them. No. Why then could I feel hay on my head? It slowly dawned on me that alas and alack the hay on my head was my fucking hair, as dry and brittle as sun baked corn. I have vowed to slather it with deep conditioning cream, but who has the time for all that shit? It's a hard enough job keeping hair off me without looking after the stuff I want to keep.

The other day I was wearing flip flops and I thought I had three white scratches on my foot. I didn't remember doing anything to scratch myself so I bent down for a closer look. The 'scratches' were in fact three cheeky bastard white hairs growing in the middle of my foot. Like a yeti! They had got long enough to fold over and lie flat against my foot, hence the confusion about scratches. I was mortified. My feet are hairy, I moaned to my gin and tonic. Something else to shave or pluck. Why is hair coming out of everywhere? What is it about my menopause that makes my body want to sprout hair ON MY FEET?

It's not as if I get cold anymore thanks to hot flushes, yet here I am with a rouge eyebrow hair that grows by stealth and then unfurls itself in public to approximately 3" long, nice and white so it stands out, lovely, glossy, dark hair bursting from my nostrils, I appear to be growing a beard, I've got hair racing out of my right armpit at a rate of knots, ditto right nipple, a biff bush that would make a 70's porn star blush, and now, hairy feet.

So please, if you are reading this and can relate, please remember you are not alone. The menopause is a fucking outrage, slowly stripping away our femininity until we are hot, hairy, pissy and slightly chubby replicas of ourselves. No wonder we have mood swings! But we can fight back. Buy that lovely make up, buy those gorgeous shoes, embrace your new curves, purchase every hair removing device you can get your hands on, treat yourself, laugh loudly (advisable to wear a piss pad though) with your friends and say Fuck you menopause. Then get up out of your chair and, because you just can't help it, fart.

Butterfly Wings
Wednesday 17th June 2020

I was talking a lovely lady the other day, this lady is just about the sweetest, kindest person you could meet, but she was feeling a bit down having had words with her teenage daughter.

Having had two such delights myself (now really lovely young ladies of whom I am immensely proud) I could sympathise by the bucketful.

Why is it that as our daughters emerge from their childhood chrysalis into beautiful beings, so gorgeous and stunning you can hardly believe such perfection came out of your flaps, our own wings start to fade and curl and dry up so much that you are more hairy brown moth than butterfly?

The smaller their knickers get the bigger mine get. It is like yin and yang. Nothing rubs salt in the cold reality of ageing quite like having two slender, striking girls in the house as you are trying to heft your flab out of the way to scrape a razor over your pubic hair which has decided, rather inexplicably, that it simply must grow down your thighs. Whatever size knickers I wear I will have a fine collection of spiders legs crawling out from the elastic. Unless I wear cycling shorts but even then, I wouldn't put money on it.

And yet, even though my body has changed beyond recognition I have a new found confidence not there before.

I like myself. I might not have the best body but I'm happy to wear what I like and fuck you, frankly, if you don't like it.

If I could go back in time and talk to my 19-year-old self I would say 'In 30 years time you will look in a mirror and be alarmed at your waistline and beard, but you won't give a shit and you need to live your life remembering that. End that crappy relationship sooner, go on fabulous holidays with your friends, cherish your grandparents, fall madly in love even though your heart will break - you will get over it, dance and laugh, give the boss who will feel you up a right good slap and march out of that awful job with your head held high, fall in love, get married, have babies, you will get fat and get hairy, but boy, will you laugh and be happy'

I've just read that back and I perhaps don't need to time travel to give myself a pep talk after all. The crappy relationship got ended. I did go on fantastic holidays with my friends (still do) I adored my grandparents, I fell madly, helplessly in love, my heart broke but I did get over it, I love to dance even though I look like I am being electrocuted, I did proper slap that twat boss with roving hands, I did march out of several awful jobs with my head held high, I fell in love at first sight with husband and would've married him later that day if it was possible. I had my children, I got fat, I got hairy but boy, do I laugh and my God, am I happy.

To all the lovely teenage daughters out there - fly high and rule the world. And to the mum's - this is to remind you that you are not a dusty old hairy moth. There are other wings besides those attached to Always piss pads and every now and then we older girls need to be reminded to give ours a shake and shine and shimmy.

The Blue Snake

Wednesday 10th June 2020

I am feeling ashamed of myself this morning.

I got dressed for work and decided to wear a nice dress (blue) and a little lime green cardigan. I put my sucky in pants on, had my legs out (fake tanned to fuck, and newly shaved) and some sparkly shoes on. Off I toddled, husband said I looked nice and I felt fabulous, sexy and ready to rule the world.

Bollocks to the menopause!

Alas, by the time I got to work a blue, knobbly snake had appeared on my lower left leg, just under the skin.

I tried to ignore it.

The snake didn't like being ignored and grew bluer and larger and more knobbly and looked like it would burst out of my fake tanned leg.

'Fuck off snake' I said. 'I will wear this dress and have my bare legs out and not let you bother me' 'Bastard'

The snake got angry. It started to pulsate with fury and engorged itself so that it wound round the back of my calf, across my shin and down to my ankle. It started to hurt.

I hobbled over to the filing cabinet feeling about as sexy as a dose of genital warts.

At half past 10 I looked down at my leg in despair and gave up. I just couldn't cope with seeing that, awful, alive, varicose vein, growing and throbbing.

Fucking menopause, I thought, I can't even feel sexy long enough for bloody pop master to start.

I rang poor husband, on his day off, and asked him to bring in some jeans and a top.

'I was just about to start strimming'

'My leg has a big blue snake on it' I sobbed

'Rubbish! I thought you looked really nice, no need to change'

'What colour dress am I wearing?' I asked.

Husband knew he was beaten.

He sounded panicked.

'What Jeans?'

'Any'

'What top?'

'Nothing see through'

Bless him and love him he arrived with a change of clothes and took my dress and lime green cardigan away.

I appeared from the toilet, happily dressed in white jeans and a blue and white top.

Mr K, my work colleague chatted to husband and asked what he was doing in the office on his day off.

'Sarah wanted to change' said husband

'Have you changed?' said Mr K in surprise.

Typical man.

I started to feel shame. There I was fretting about an admittedly horrid varicose vein crawling up my leg, thinking the whole world would see it and think urgh. When in fact the only person who was bothered abut it was me.

I became so fixated on it that I made my husband come in on his day off with a change of clothes for me.

For feck's sake, I made my husband go through my wardrobe and exposed him to all my new clothes, completely voiding my 'Oh, but I've had this thing for ages' argument because half the stuff in there still has fucking labels on.

If one of my friends had done this, I would've said they looked gorgeous, nobody else is bothered, don't be silly, you are a proud, strong woman etc etc, but I could not apply this kindness to myself. Quicker than you can say 'double chin' I put my blue knobbly leg inside my jeans and hid the bastard thing.

But as least I still have my sparkly shoes on. Closed toes of course. Nobody likes a hairy toe.

I Am Still Me
30th June 2020

I've no idea what has prompted this, perhaps it was the news this morning, that a sexual predator was released 'by mistake' from prison to go on a rampage of rape and abuse again. And that the powers that be are sorry that this mistake happened. One of his 'mistakes' was a 71-year-old lady. Perhaps this angered me so much that I wanted to tell my story.

So today (deep breath) I am going to write about something deeply personal to me. I was sexually abused as an 8-year-old by the headmaster at my Primary school. He chose his target well, I was new to the school, a protective old sister recently moved into an inexperienced teacher's class. I mention my sibling because he threatened her as collateral, I suppose, in case I said anything. He need not have worried. In the 1970's those of us who were being abused had no voice, there quite literally were no words to say what was happening to us because the words did not exist.

I tried to speak without using words. I went to the hairdresser and made them cut my hair short. 'I want to look like a boy' In my childish mind if I looked like a boy, he would leave me alone.

Into the class he came and looked around, with his fleshy, jowly face and lascivious leer. He did not recognise me. It had worked. Elation soared inside me as the terror subsided. He leant over and asked the teacher where I was. She pointed me out. That betrayal stings to this day. But she did not know. Young herself and in her first teaching job, she simply smiled and gave me to him. Nowadays alarm bells would scream the place down. But not back then. He used the guise of swimming lessons to conduct his abuse. Week in and week out I had to leave the class, walk out of where I should be safe and into his lair, the changing room; a wooden chalet detached from the school building.

I tried to speak the words that didn't exist by pulling my eyelashes out. Hospital visits to poke and prod at my eyelids 'silly girl doing this to yourself' eventually it was put down to a nervous habit. No shit Sherlock. Now hair pulling is recognised as a sign of reaction to extreme stress. I wish I could go back in time and put my arms around that little girl and tell her that what she is doing is her way of asking for help. I would tell her there is so much pain inside her that she is doing her best to release it. She need not feel the scalding shame that she will carry around for so many years. It is not her shame to feel. It is his. It won't make any difference. She will feel shame regardless.

I would tell her that she will soon learn to bury the memory of what is happening. The headmaster will shortly retire and a new one, kind and decent will save her by restoring her faith in school. I will tell her that she will bury the memory so deep she will be able to have a normal life for a while. The flashbacks and nightmares will come later.

If sexual abuse were a physical injury, it would be a raw, open, throbbing, angry gaping wound stretched the length of your body and cut down to the bone. Often times there are no obvious physical signs which is why so may turn to self-abuse. You must have a release valve for the pain.

Why am I telling my story now? Because 40 years on I am what I am because of what that little girl went through. The monster is long dead. But I am alive. I may suffer nightmares and flashbacks, the smell of wet creosote (the changing rooms were coated in it) makes me shudder with revulsion, but I get through it. I have learnt to love myself. Some days I have to reach deep down inside me to find the strength to face the day. I leave the room when people start talking about sexual abuse cases in the news. I simply cannot listen. I am stronger and I am weaker. I am harder and I am kinder. I will stop and chat to rough sleepers because, there but for the grace of God, go I.

I have learnt the value of words. Through this page I communicate the frustrations and tribulations of middle age. I have found my voice at long last, and today feels like the right time to tell the story of a little girl. My story. It is a story I have told to only a handful of people throughout my life. The fear of rejection because people don't know what to say has kept me quiet. But I finally have the words I was denied as a child.

To everyone who has told their story before me, thank you for your bravery. You have opened doors that didn't even exist 40 years ago. I am not a victim I am a survivor. And my God, I am proud of myself. The shame never quite leaves you. But I want you to know who I am. I am strong. I am a survivor. I'm OK. I'm still me.

To anyone going through this, please use your voice to ask for the help you deserve. You are not alone. You are NOT alone.

How to Know When You Are Middle Aged
Monday 20th July 2020

Your mind turns to mush and you can't remember why you went into a room (unless it's the toilet, then it's run, drop the goods and be thankful you got there in time).

Your nose is hairy.

Laughing and sneezing are directly connected to your pelvic floor. It's like being at the fairground 'the louder you scream the faster we go' only now it's the louder you sneeze the faster the flow.

You develop a sixth sense for when that big grey eyebrow hair is ready to be plucked and can get it without using a mirror.

Half your life is spent pulling granny bristles out of your chin. Just when you think you've got them all you grow another fecking chin.

You really start to like Gin. Tonic optional.

You cannot apply mascara without opening your mouth. If you close your mouth you end up squinting.

Your knickers are approximately the same size as your pillow case.

Elastic waists are no longer just for granny; they are a selling point.

You start collecting random bits of crockery.

1986 was only 20 years ago.

You haven't seen your belly button for 18 months.

You have five grey barbed wire pubic hairs.

You say the following on a regular basis:

These bathroom scales are fucking shit.

I will lose a stone by Easter/Summer/Christmas.

This is the last time I'm having a takeaway.

Gin and tonic has less calories than a banana.

My jeans have shrunk in the wash.

Miracle youth serum my arse.

What time is Countryfile on?

Why is my phone in the fridge?

Am I the only person who cleans this fecking house?

Pass the Febreze, I've just pissed a bit.

And finally, finally, after a very long time, you have learnt not to give too much of a shit what other people think of you, and it feels quite marvellous.

Skopelos

16th August 2020

Today I have bagged myself a sea front sun bed. After a day on holiday, I've just changed colour from white to red and blotchy, have spent the night with mosquito's feeding on my arse and have decided I am are brave enough to wear a tankini today, the better to show off my bites and sunburn.

The beach is shingle so I have purchased some attractive beach shoes to wear on land and in the sea. I look like I have club feet. Alas for my ego, a beautiful, younger, slender, perfectly golden girl has rocked up on the fucking sun bed next to me. Bitch!

There's a whole row of empty sunbeds to go at. She has glided over the shingle with perfectly polished toe nails. No ugly beach shoes for this goddess. Just to further decimate my body confidence she keeps turning her peachy thong clad bum in my direction.

And yes, she's opening those legs wide to make sure her firm thighs get bronzed to perfection.

I'll just have a quick check that I snipped all my spiders' legs off, tuck a flopped-out flap in and strike the same pose myself. We could be twins!

Sod it love, you'll be like me in about 25 years! Such is the life of a middle-aged woman on holiday. Pass me a cocktail, it's 5pm somewhere.

The Nudists

7th October 2020

Just back off a lovely sunny Greek holiday with the husband. Just the two of us in a villa booked last minute. Nice and private. Very private. Private enough for a spot of first time nude sunbathing. No kids around to vomit at the state of us. Out came the sun, up went the temperature and off came the clothes. Sun cream was carefully and thoroughly applied to those bits where no sun has gone before. We positioned ourselves so that there was no way next door could possibly see us unless they hung out of their window by their ankles, bent their body to a right angle and used a periscope, and, trust me, the sight to see was not worth the risk.

We basked in the sun, bums facing up to the sky. It was very liberating. But nobody wants a crispy arse so we had to turn over. We basked in the sun once more. My boobs spread out nicely under each arm pit and full on fanny exposure. Husband's lad and plums were ripe for the taking. We relaxed, I opened up my legs - the better to do the inside thigh, and husband spread out - the better to do his bollocks - when all of a sudden we heard 'yoo hoo' over the fecking fence. But wait! The fence is nice and high and nobody can see over unless they are on stilts. Our blood froze in the blistering heat. Where was this fucking yoo hoo-ing coming from? Who on earth could possibly see us? Alas, there is a locked gate cut into the fence which has a visible small narrow slot (not the only visible slot in the garden that day) at eye level and through which the villa owner was peering through, eyes bleeding at the sight of us. You have never seen anybody move so quick. Husband had a towel round him quicker than you can say 'Fuck, my flaps are out!' which is, coincidently, exactly what I did say.

I grabbed a floaty chiffon sarong which concealed absolutely nothing, squared my shoulders and prepared to have a conversation with a man who had just seen straight up me and almost out the other side. Husband opened up the gate and let the poor man in.

I don't get embarrassed easily but my face burnt and flamed that day and not from the sun.

To be fair he should have let us know what time he was going to call round, but perhaps he felt that a boring, middle aged couple would be a safe bet to visit on the first full day of their holiday. Maybe he thought we would be dressed in tweed, taking tea, listening to Ken Bruce and discussing political matters, not sprawled out knob and flaps first drinking beer by the gallon.

You live and learn Mr villa owner. Underestimate the British middle aged man and woman at your peril. Hope your eyes are better now, bleach might help.

The Giant Poodle in the Bath
13th October 2020

Last night I had that rare treat – a bubble bath. To make sure my body was fully submerged and concealed in case - horrors! – anyone should come in and see me in the raw, I put as much Radox in as I could get away with. The bathroom lathered up like a flood in a washing powder factory. All that was visible were my eyes peeking out through a bouffant of bubbles, which was perfect as far as I was concerned.

I settled down into the water and ordered my head to relax.

Alas, the dogs wanted to join me in the bathroom. Dennis was especially astonished that I had seemingly turned myself into a giant white poodle and barked loudly right in my ear.

'Feck off Dennis' I said, lovingly. Bark, Bark, Bark, Bark went the little gobshite, getting more and more outraged. This was not relaxing in anyway shape or form.

I was rescued by my daughter who tempted Dennis away with a biscuit, all thoughts of his beloved mummy being consumed by a poodle suddenly vanished from his empty little head.

I tried to relax again. Harry, our other dog, a chocolate lab who is older and much wiser than Dennis, rolled his eyes at such foolishness and lay down on the floor. His bum nudged one of the drawers on the bathroom cabinet which let out a little squeak. Harry jumped up whining and barking and turning round and round in circles trying to eat the squeak. At last, Harry decided this was a stupid waste of energy and thought to settle himself on my dressing gown which I had carefully thrown in a heap on the floor.

I tried to read my book but couldn't see through the wall of bubbles. I lay back and finally started to switch off. The heat from the bath had relaxed my stomach a bit too much and I let out an avalanche of farts, one of them dangerous which made me think it was time to get out. I heaved myself out of the bath, morphed from poodle to overweight middle-aged woman with an excessive wind problem and looked in the mirror. My face was red and my moustache was blonde. I looked like a 1970's German porno star, minus, thankfully, the penis. I think I preferred looking like a monstrous, mutant poodle. Daughter came to my rescue again with some wax strips. They had a pretty, innocent looking daisy on the packaging, implying that the product was nice and natural, gentle, soothing and calming, blah blah bullshit. The fucking things nearly took my top lip off. I howled with pain and instinctively dabbed my still sticky red raw lip with my dressing gown. Which was covered in dark brown chocolate Labrador hair. From middle aged woman to poodle to German porn star to Tom fucking Sellek.

I guess it just wasn't my night.

I Chose Bridgerton
January 11th 2021

So, the year got off to a fantastic start when I developed a slight cold (not Corona) and I kept sneezing. Violently. As anybody who has to drag their pelvic floor along on the ground behind them will know, sneezes are terrible things.

On one fabulous day I sneezed twice in the kitchen and my piss pad just threw its little wings up in the air and said 'I'm no fucking match for that' curled up and died. Off I dashed to the loo. Followed by a dash to the bedroom for a change of clothes, and a bigger pad. All fresh and lovely. I sneezed again. I squeezed my legs shut. Safe. Phew. But then along came another sneeze. Followed by an inexplicable torrent, considering I had just been to the bastard toilet. Large piss pad said 'Fuck me, I'm drowning' and gave up. I stripped off again and, starkers from the waist down, began to inch my way to the loo once more.

I have to go down a flight of stairs to get to the loo. At the top of the stairs, I sneezed again. I tried to keep it in, but I felt the trickle. 'This is fucking outrageous!' I screamed to absolutely nobody. I looked around for something to help me make it to the loo without leaving a piss trail. Option 1, my new fleecy pyjama top. Option 2, husbands beloved England rugby top.

I think we all know how this ends, but fair to say, England's Rose had a generous watering, I found my ginormous piss knickers and, finally, all was calm.

The next day I got out of bed and farted. I farted as I stood up. I farted as I bent down to get my dressing gown. I farted as I walked round the bed. 'Is it going to stop?' asked husband. 'I don't know' was the honest reply. I farted myself down the stairs and farted myself round the rest of the house. Reach up for a coffee cup. Fart. Bend down to put spoon in dishwasher. Fart. Drink Coffee. Fart. It was, even by my standards, quite astonishing. I think that the gas had been forced to back up in my vast piss knickers, and, when I was finally able remove them, we had blast off.

All this pissing and farting made me feel quite unladylike and, with the added bonus of another lockdown, which means we have had to cancel a holiday (booked back in 2019) for Husband's 60th, it is fair to say I was a little bit down. To cheer myself up I trawled through Netflix looking for a box set.

I chose Bridgerton. Oh, be still my beating heart, which lies under several layers of floppy, occasionally quite hairy bosom. My eyes have literally seen the coming of the Lord (or the Duke of Hastings) and I am left with an uncontrollable urge to want to sink my teeth into his rather fine arse.

If you haven't watched Bridgerton, on Netflix, put it on now. You will need a fan because a hot flush is NOTHING compared to what you will experience whilst watching certain episodes. You may feel swoony at certain points. If you watch it with your 19- and 18-year-old daughters, as I did, you will wish you had never been born, and, no doubt, your children will wish they had never been born either. You will feel mortification actually crawling along your skin and shame bursting out from every pore. But none of you will be able to take your eyes from the screen and you will be glued to that lovely bottom going up and down and in and out like the clappers.

The gloom and doom of 2021 suddenly felt very, very far away and for that Bridgerton is to be cheered to the rafters.

Most Said Phrases of 2021 (Already)
13th January 2021

For Fucks sake (rolled over from 2020)

No

Because it's lockdown

Mum the internet isn't working

Turn it off and turn it on again

I'm not Bill Bastard Gates

Unplug it and plug it back in again.

Jesus! Throw the sodding thing out of the window.

Count yourself lucky to have the internet.

In my day we had to go to the library.

In my day we used a microfiche

I can't be arsed to explain.

Lockdown won't last for ever.

Will it?

What day is it?

Where has all the food gone?

The fecking fridge was full yesterday!

I'm going to book an Asda delivery

Fuckers! There are no slots available

I'm going to book a click and collect.

Fuckers! There are no slots available.

Pass the Gin

Lockdown Day 297
Thursday 14th January 2021

There is a box on the top right of the Daily Mail online which states today is Lockdown Day 297. I don't know why but this got me thinking. 297 days of my life have gone by! And what have I accomplished?

I tried Joe Wicks and thought he was a lovely chap, but bouncing around doing the kangaroo hops with piss leaking out of me like a skunk spraying scent, well, it wasn't for me.

I tried online yoga. I love yoga. But the internet connection in our house is so shite that I was often left in a particularly awkward pose with my head much closer to my crotch than I would like without realising that the screen had frozen and I could've removed my nose from my flaps five minutes previously.

I tried to lose weight. Christ, after 297 days I thought I'd be to be as slinky as a racing snake. My clothes should be hanging off me. But somewhere along the line I just couldn't be fucking bothered with all that and drank Gin and ate crisps instead.

I really tried to keep up a personal grooming routine, but fuck me sideways, life is surely too short. Eyebrows, nose, moustache, chin, pits, nips, pubes (endless battle ground) legs and, finally, toes. I swear there is not a part of me where hair will not grow. I went a bit feral at one point until husband (also quite hairy) and I got stuck together like Velcro.

I tried to improve my education by learning another language and downloaded an App to upgrade my basic French from 'Je voudrais une grande bière s'il vous plaît'

to a level where I could at least hold a conversation, albeit aided by wildly extravagant hand gestures. But I'll be honest with you, I found myself reading crap stories in Take a Break instead and thanking the powers that be that Google translate exists for lazy fuckers like me.

So, in 297 days I have sprayed my living room rug with piss whilst pretending to be a kangaroo, sniffed my own crotch for longer than I thought possible, drank gallons of Gin, got fatter, gone yeti and enjoyed reading about somebody's dirty bastard husband stuffing the next-door neighbour as well as the turkey.

It's a funny old life.

The Knicker Drawer
Wednesday 20th January 2021

It is raining. It is January. My holiday has been cancelled. We are in sodding lockdown. Everything is a little bit shit, but! I am going to focus on the positives. At least now that my beach break has been kiboshed, I can slack off on the never ending and, frankly thankless, daily battle to calm down my pubic hair long enough to trim it into a manageable style that can be tucked into a swimming costume. Free the fandango hair! It can now revert to its default state of knee length wire wool and I can scare the poor therapist to death when I go in for a wax at some distant point in the future. She will probably think I've got a big brown poodle on my lap. Or a newfoundland.

I can use lockdown to sort out all the crap we have accumulated and stuffed in various cupboards and drawers around our house. Or, I can use lockdown to do a blind tasting of all the lovely Gins I have accumulated every time I go to Aldi. And then I won't give a shit about my cupboards of crap.

I can sort my underwear drawer out which is in a shameful state. No other word for it. There are layers and layers of knickers telling the story of my life. Buried at the bottom we have the slinky, minxy size 12 going-on-a-date and might-get-a-ride thongs of yesteryear.

Layer two. The slightly more practical I'm- engaged-or-married-now-so-fuck-off-wearing-a-thong knickers; still skimpy and, compared to now, tiny, and kept just in case I run out of hankies.

Layer three. An increase in size to 12-14 here we have the very worn, a little bit grey and a little bit stretched with the occasional hole in them (sadly for husband, not in the crotch) everyday pants that withered and died and gave up and told me to fuck off trying to cram my arse in them as I got bigger.

Layer four. Size 14. Lacy and black in a desperate attempt to look sexy but comfy and big enough to be pulled up over the stomach. Wide enough to accommodate the new, must have, knicker accessory - the piss pad.

Top layer. Size 16! Massive, fucking awful granny pants that could sail a fucking ship! They come up nice and high to give the illusion of wobble smoothing, but, the minute you step outside, they fall down just enough for a roll of flab to protrude over the top. You hate them. Also on the top layer of the drawer, but squashed in towards the back so you can pretend that you don't own them, are actual fat sucker in pants that look like cycling shorts, they are so tight that they are near impossible to get on. It is exhausting. They vacuum pack the air out of your lungs so that you are puce and sweating and collapsed on the bed remembering why the bastard things have been shoved at the back of the drawer in the first place. They squish the flab up and down so that it bulges out at your armpits and knees and are about as sexy as a dose of the clap.

On second thoughts, I think I will make a nice cup of tea and pluck my chin instead.

The Black Sea
5th February 2022

I should put a warning on this post that it does describe how the menopause can make you feel. It is not a pretty read, but shit happens.

I woke up one morning a few weeks ago feeling, as usual, fat, floppy, tired, shit and pissed off that I had not lost four stone overnight.

The menopause has been unkind to me in many ways; I have gained weight and facial hair. I am forgetful, hormonal, moody and a raging insomniac. I used to feel so capable and organised, and yet now, at times, I am a distracted, absent-minded version of myself who I barely recognise. I feel very emotional, tears are often not very far away and laughter feels like something I have to force up and out.

Other times I feel a burning rage when somebody is talking; People chewing, and even breathing can drive me to a murderous rage.

I should have shares in KY jelly and Tena Lady. Nobody talks enough about all the crap that happen to us.

And yet, the menopause has also given me confidence that I could only have dreamt of in my 20's. I don't give much of a shit what people think of me. I am lucky enough to have a close group of friends who I would go to the stake for, I love my family and adore my husband. Everything else is a bonus.

However, three weeks ago I could not shake the feeling that I have to start making a change. I don't like feeling like a blob. I am 50 this summer and would like to be at least a size smaller and more toned. I don't want back fat or a saddle bag roll where my stomach drags down. My new found confidence does not extend to my body. I don't like looking in the mirror. I see only flaws. It makes me sad.

I love yoga, but our studio has closed down due to Covid. And I love belly dancing, it is balm on my soul, however yoga and belly dancing are all on line now and our Wi-Fi is so bad at home that zoom things are impossible.

I found myself slipping back towards depression, everyone has a different way of describing depression: black dog, black wave etc, for me it is a black sea, thankfully it is usually far off on the horizon, but always there. At times it has crept up on me and before I know it, I am submerged, lost, and it takes other people and pills to help me out. Now I have learnt to recognise the signs, the black sea was pooling round my ankles, I wanted to fight back.

So, waking up three weeks ago I turned my head and eyed up the treadmill that my husband has in his gym area. I fucking hate running. It hurts. But, almost in a trance, I downloaded the couch to 5k app, pulled on my, now redundant, yoga pants and slouched over to the running machine.

The couch to 5k starts off gently, walk, run, walk etc. I wobbled and blobbed and sobbed and felt ridiculous. I had pain in my legs and I loathed every second, but I finished day one and crawled to the shower to wash off all the sweat. You go back to the app every other day. I am just about to start week 4 and to my astonishment I have kept at it. I still fucking hate it, I really hate it, but I am proud of myself for having a go. And the black sea is back on the horizon where it can fucking well stay, thank you very much.

I have not suddenly shrunk in size and I still look like a jelly on a trampoline, I won't win any awards for running, but at least I am honest about the shit we have to go through when our bodies and minds undergo this most unwelcome, intrusive change, and I am finally facing up to the fact that only I can do something about altering my fitness if I want to.

Every other morning for the foreseeable future, I will be collapsed in a heap, using whatever breath I can muster, to call the treadmill a cock dick bastard bell end twat. Somethings will never change.

So, to anybody out there having a bad day - keep going. We are not only coping with the pandemic and all the shit, grief and horror it brings, we are also battling the menopause – and, from somewhere deep down inside, we are finding the strength to stick two fingers up to it and laugh at ourselves. You are brilliant. Keep fighting.

The Elixir

11th February 2021 - Lockdown day 3689

Do you know, about 2 years ago, I actually went in to a House of Fraser department store, and asked the lovely assistant at the Clinique section to sell me something that would give me a dewy, youthful glow? I said it confidently and in all seriousness. The poor 20-year-old assistant – herself no stranger to excessive lip liner – looked as if I had asked if she would mind very much if I twisted out a shit on her counter. Her eyes widened in panic as she took in my middle-aged face. I stood there patiently, feeling genuinely excited and confident that such a product existed.

Lots of serums and moisturisers were procured, and I agreed to an in-store makeover. I had plucked my chin and nostrils that morning so it was safe to expose my upturned face in public. Approximately £10,000 worth of lotions, potions and make up were applied to my head and I came out with a dent in my bank balance and an alarmingly orange face. The minute I got home I wiped it all off and put my usual slap back on.

I don't know what madness came over me thinking there was a magical elixir that can wipe the years from your face. Yes, you can have Botox and fillers and face lifts, and if that is your thing then good luck to you. But it must be hard to stop tampering and let nature take its course, so you keep on filling and plumping and lifting and freezing until you look vaguely alien.

I think we need to celebrate aging and the changes that happen to us. It is not a crime to grow old and, although it is hard to accept the changes that happen – that Mother Nature has an awful cruel streak, the bitch. I don't need chin hair or an 18-inch special grey eyebrow hair thank you very much. I don't need to piss myself when I jump or sneeze either. Or fart when I bend over.

From here on in, I am going to be more positive and try to accept that my face and body are changing, perhaps not for the better if we judge only on youthful skin and slender firm bodies, but they are changing anyway and there isn't much I can do about it.

I don't think age is celebrated enough. Every one of my lines around my eyes are there because I have thrown my head back and roared with laughter. My skin is aging because I have spent happy days in the sun squinting as I watch my children play on holiday whilst sipping a big fuck off cocktail. I am larger than I would like to be because I have enjoyed fabulous food and one too many drinks and have not moved my arse enough to counter this.

My husband promises that he has a special cure all, that will make me thinner and younger. I can take it orally or rub it over my face or chest. The magic potion is not fussy as to how or where it is applied but would work better if taken at least 6 times a day.

Despite my husband's assurances, there is no magic potion to make us younger, but a fabulous haircut, a bit of sun on our skin and a visit to the spa can do the world of good. So, unless this country wants to see a middle aged, menopausal revolution, I suggest they think about opening hairdressers, salons and spas pretty quickly. And the pub! Otherwise, a load of cranky women with awful roots, overgrown fanny hair, beards and droopy grey faces will descend on parliament. I'll bring the Gin.

Narky, old, hairy and pissed? They'll think we are all MP's.

Sudocrem Vs Valentine's Day
Tuesday 16th February 2021

Ah, valentines' day has been and gone. I hope yours fared better than mine.

Husband had got me chocolates, flowers and cards and I had got him fuck all. I hastily said I would make him a nice roast dinner which we were going to have anyway. Then inspiration struck! I would do some maintenance on the fandango foliage. Long overdue I have to admit. I fancied myself creating a nice love heart shape or maybe a little landing strip.

There was a major obstacle to this fantasy: I cannot actually see my growler to groom it because my tummy is in the way. So, I snipped vaguely and carefully around my neither region with the scissors.

I realise I could've stood up, hefted up my roll and looked in the mirror but I would have to bleach my eyeballs for the next five years, and it is not worth it, frankly.

I soon gave up on the love heart shape, it resembled Africa, if anything – massively impressive if my husband was a geography teacher - but he is an estate agent. So, I went for the landing strip.

The landing strip had bald spots in it. In fact, once I had given the old girl a severe cut, I realised it was alarmingly sparse in places. A patch here and a patch there. Not very sexy. So, I got out my razor and sheared the lot off.

I cleaned the bath (2 hours and 1 bin bag) and slipped into something sexy. The least I could do, having ignored Valentine's Day, was to not wear dishcloth grey saggy arsed pants.

I went into our Artic bedroom and put on the electric blanket. Husband had received a coded message via text (sex?) so I knew he would be up soon.

I lay down seductively.

My newly bald fanny started to burn a little bit.

I won't lie, this was quite nice at first because our room is very cold and my normally abundant hair keeps me warm around the flap area. But soon it started really burning and itching.

I wriggled around on the bed and tried to scratch it with the duvet.

Burn, burn, burn, itch, itch, itch.

I spied some Sudocrem, probably last used on my babies bottoms in 2003, and pounced on it like it was a £50.00 note that husband had left lying around.

I slathered it on everywhere that was itching. It was blissfully calming and the itchy burning soothed.

I tried to rub it in a bit more so that my entire mid-section looked less like an explosion in a Tippex factory. The more

I rubbed the less it went in. It just smeared itself further around my body. I rubbed my face in exasperation, Sudocrem was now multiplying on my cheeks. Fucks Sake! What is in that stuff? The burning started again. The fan looked very inviting. I tried to wipe my hands on my arse cheeks, the logic being there was ample flesh there to soak up the wretched stuff, before turning on the fan

So, there I was, two white handprints on my arse, Sudocrem on 90% of my body aiming the fan at my glowing, balding, blindingly white fanny which looked for all the world like freshly plucked chicken skin dipped in correction fluid, when husband appeared.

Lights off it is then, Said Mr Romance.

Insomnia
Friday 19th February 2021

Another marvellous night of insomnia last night.

It went like this: 10.45 to 11 pm. Take Night Nurse, go to bed, read for a bit, chatter to husband. He starts talking about some boring car part or needing a new razor because his is somehow stuffed with pubes, it's a fecking Glillete Mach 3 if I don't mind and can I remember that he has to use it on his fecking face next time I feel like landscaping and did I realise I was going grey blah blah blah, I tune out and fall asleep.

Wake up at 1.03 am I am wide awake. Why? It is the middle of the fucking night.

At 1.15 am I put my sleep app on and play a nice little story with a soothing voice. It lasts 45 minutes and I have never heard the end of it. I always drift off before getting to the end.

Sometime between 1.15 and 2.45 am Fall asleep.

2.45 am Husband gets up for a wee. Stumbles around bumping into things as if the fecker is deliberately trying to wake me up. Leaves the room. I fall asleep.

2.48 am Husband comes back in the room, crashes around in the dark like a fucking drunken sailor on shore leave, ricochets off every wall and every surface as if he is suddenly one legged and blind. Succeeds in waking me up.

He gets in to bed and is instantly deeply asleep, despite my narrowed eyeballs boring into him. With extra venom.

2.48 to 3.15am Toss and turn and huff and puff in a vain attempt to wake husband up who now appears to be deaf and comatose.

3.15 am Give up trying to wake husband and put sleep app back on. Select the fire crackle sounds, gentle crickets chirping and soft bird singing to lull me to sleep.

3.37 am App is shit. Fucking crickets getting on my tits.

3.38 am Put sleep app story back on.

3.45 am Eyes feel heavy nearly asleep.

4.45 am Husband wakes me up from blissful deep sleep to ask if I heard the fucking dog barking.

4.46 am Husband instantly back in a deep sleep leaving me glaring at him with pure hate.

4.46 to 5 am Contemplate stabbing him with my nose hair scissors but too much faff to wash the bedding afterwards.

5 to 6:15 am Wide awake. Can actually feel my stubble growing.

6.20 am Fall asleep.

6.45 am Alarm goes off. Husband full of beans after a wonderful nights sleep. Fancies himself getting the ride. Is told to shove it up his own hairy hole.

6.45 to 7.15 am Lie there with mad unblinking staring eyes, literally unable to believe that I have to summon the energy to get up.

7.15 am Fart and a bit of wee comes out too. Panic. Fart myself out of bed and stumble to the loo.

7.25 am Think I nodded off on the loo, come to with a jolt and am astonished to find I am still pissing. It's been 10 minutes. How is this possible? Am I a race horse?

And so, another day begins.

The End (Of Lockdown) Is Nigh
Tuesday 23rd February 2021

So, after I discovered that I really cannot run, my couch to 5k has been slightly downgraded to very fast walking. I walk like there is a fire behind my arse just about to singe the undercarriage, or as if someone is dangling a bottle of gin just out of reach in front of me. It's a waddle wobble walk but I'm getting off my arse most days to do it. Naturally, I expected instant weight loss and naturally, after one walk, I was crushed with disappointment to find I had stayed exactly the same. I walked past a photo of me on my wedding day on the way to the bathroom scales. How slim I looked! The only thing that still fits me now from my wedding day are my fucking earrings.

But I have had two children. I have eaten and drunk some very lovely things over the years and I have got middle aged. The spread arrived quite gradually. I always thought it was a myth, this middle-aged spread, something fat people used as an excuse. But now I am the fat person using it as an excuse and I find it is perfectly reasonable to do so. I have got bigger as I've got older. It's quite a comfort, having a roll to rest your arms on. It keeps me warm. I used to blame the fact that I had just had two babies in quick succession but they are 19 and 18 now, so that doesn't really wash. Plus, HRH Catherine has popped three out and is slimmer than the lower part of my leg so I can't really use childbirth to justify my wobble.

It would be OK if everyone around me was the same, but alas, alas, two good friends have lost weight over the lockdowns and now look slim and trim and fit. And I look like a blonde Ma Larkin. With 6 inches of dark brown roots.

Even husband has lost weight by having Granola every day. Rabbit hutch scrapings! I just cannot bring myself to eat it.

But now, we have an incentive......lockdown is ending, at least we think it is, nobody is really sure......and I would like to face my long-lost loved ones with a new slimmer figure. They will say 'Wow! Where have you gone?' instead of 'Oh! I do love your elasticated leggings' My awful, vile giant, massive sleep two tent Spanx pants will be on the bonfire along with, I hope, my face mask. I will wear skimpy underwear and I will see my growler for the first time since 2001. I will check to see if I still have a belly button. Does it go in or out? I can't remember. I haven't seen the fucking thing for years. I will be able to shave my legs without lifting my belly out of the way. I will eat nothing but salad and fruit until I can shit through the eye of a needle and I will lose my muffin top and bingo wings. I will walk as fast and as furiously as I can every day and I WILL LOSE WEIGHT.

And then, when lock down ends, I will go to every restaurant and pub I can fucking well find and put it all back on again. With a smile on my big fat face.

Normal life, look out, I am coming for you. I've missed you; it's been far too long.

Lockdown Madness
Thursday 25th March 2021

And so, another week draws to a close, life is like fucking Groundhog Day.

I only realised how crap everything had become when my 19-year-old daughter – a second year university student who, let's be honest, should be face down in a Wetherspoons somewhere – got excited about coming to Morrison's with me.

What have we done to our kids?

My life has been an exciting whirlwind these last few days. Try to keep up as I take you on a nonstop tour of high drama. First, we had the dizzy heights of date night with husband in Sainsbury's car park (another supermarket! Am obviously a supermarket whore) which involved a ready mixed can of G & T, Take and Break and a packet of Quavers, and no head bobbing activity much to husband's disappointment. As if one can of ready mixed gin and tonic would be enough, and besides, as I exclaimed at the time: 'It's Sainsbury's! not Kwik Save!'

I had a toilet experience during which I appeared to shit out something the length of a garden hose. It fought back against multiple flushes and skirmishes with the toilet brush and I started to sweat with fear that I wouldn't get rid of it before lockdown ends on the 12th of never and we can have visitors again. Finally, after a protracted battle, the hosepipe poo gave up left the building.

Then we had the great excitement of a visit to Homebase.

When do we go from saying 'let's go out tonight and get shit faced' to 'Let's go to Homebase and buy a new lawnmower?'

On Sunday the sun came out – hang onto your seats - and I got over excited because I could do my pots.

Yes, putting primroses into fucking pots was the pinnacle of my weekend.

Husband admired his shiny new lawnmower, which is too good to be used on the lawn apparently, so he is still using his shitty Flymo circa 1856, and I stuffed pansies and compost into clay pots and wondered when exactly it was that I turned into an old woman.

I don't want to get excited about garden centres and I don't want to waste any more of my life wondering if the pink pansy should go next to the yellow primrose. I don't want to give a shit about potted plants. I want to get pissed with my mates and dance my flaps off.

Life is now so devoid of normality that me buying three brand new baking trays for £7.50 is something our entire household, including the dogs, got excited about.

And I can't tell you the adrenaline rush when I made Mary Berry's steak and ale casserole with dumplings! It was like we had won the lottery. Lockdown lunacy has landed.

I feel like the old Sarah is trapped inside this caged shell and she is getting closer and closer to bursting out, saying Fuck it! running to the pub, grabbing a large gin, running to the hairdressers, kissing everybody and feeling normal again. So, Boris, hurry up and let us out of this madhouse, please. Don't move the goalposts, don't backtrack, don't mess with our heads. My roots are inexplicable, I have a fucking mono brow and the momma bear in me is getting very pissed off for the sake of her kids. And momma bear is a menopausal, pansy arranging, hosepipe shitting scary piece of work.

Chip Butties and Gin
24th June 2021

There has been a lot of chatter about the menopause recently, and not to take anything away from the celebrities who have been, quite rightly and refreshingly talking about it, but I have not seen or heard from anybody like me. I don't have the energy or the motivation to exercise myself into a size 6. I don't have access to a personal trainer or pots of money for lovely treatments and, maybe, one or two tweaks.

I don't keep to a strict diet. I like Wotsits and chip butties. And God, but I love a nice gin and tonic. So, whilst I applaud these ladies for talking out, seeing a fabulously fit and gorgeous celeb talking about the menopause doesn't resonate with me. Because I have a roll of flab hanging over my jeans, a droopy eyelid and a varicose vein that looks like a blue snake.

My life has been remarkably unremarkable. I am a woman who got married, raised a family and worked hard. I come home at night, knackered, and do the housework and cook the dinner. I feel taken for granted, sometimes. And I am every woman who has seen her figure widen and her face wrinkle.

Slowly, slowly age creeps in and takes over. And we don't put up much of a fight. We are too busy being busy. Until menopause.

Suddenly the shit hits the fan. You have no clue what is going on because your brain fogs up overnight. Your pelvic floor stops being able to function normally and decides it is now perfectly acceptable to leak a trail of piss wherever you go. Getting up out of an armchair now requires assistance in the form of a massive, uncontrollable fart. It takes everybody by surprise, most of all you. And the more people in the vicinity the louder the fart will be. Sometimes you have to fart your way across the room as you walk. You try to make light of it but inside you are wondering what the fuck has happened to make your arsehole flap like a pair of elephant ears on a hot day.

And the mood swings! Anger boils over and out of you like red hot lava spewing from a volcano. You are happy, you are depressed, you are laughing, you are in tears all in the space of five minutes. You adore your husband he is sweet and understanding. You hate your husband – why does he breathe so fucking loudly? You are a nympho and want sex like a sailor on shore leave. You get upstairs and feel as sexy as a 97year old nun whose fandango withered, dried up and retired long, long ago.

And somewhere in midst of this madness, the old you is looking on, aghast at the changes being wrought on your body and mind. Clothes don't fit, wrinkle creams are shit. Piss pads are a God send. It appears that, despite your best efforts, once you hit 45 you are supposed to have a beard and a moustache, a foot long grey eyebrow hair and Brillo pad pubes. If I didn't wax my chin, I could audition for ZZ top. Everybody gets on your fucking nerves. You are so tired and yet wide-awake night after night listening to your brain whirling up an anxiety storm.

It is frightening and awful and bewildering.

But it does not last forever.

So, buy the piss pads, go up a size (or two), pluck like fuck and talk about these changes. Hoof as dry as a desert in a drought? Get a tube of lube. Feel fat? Get some big suck it in pants or wear a thong, whatever. It is your party and you will find that, somewhere along the line, you stop caring about what other people think of you. The menopause is nothing to be ashamed of. It is an outrage! Before menopause I could hold a conversation at work, type an email, plan the evening meal and arrange my social life all at the same time. Now the only things I can do simultaneously are sneeze and piss. You can take up dancing, jogging, sailing, knitting whatever. Or you can just sit on your arse, like I do most of the time, and do sweet shag all. Laugh and drink Gin with your loved ones. If I can give you one last piece of advice: By all means do a parachute jump, swim with sharks, race on a motor bike but please, when wearing white jeans, don't bend over and fart. Some risks are not worth taking.

Leather Pants and Fanny Farts
Sunday September 5th 2021

Last night we went round to a friend's house and I surprisingly and rather rashly decided to wear my fake leather pants. I haven't worn them for ages and couldn't think why as, to me anyway, they looked and felt super sexy. I asked my eldest to curl my hair, put on a black top, some knee-high boots and nice make up.

I thought I looked like a fatter, older but passable version of Sandy from Grease.

Fuck it all, I was going to rock this look!

Down the stairs I squeaked and creaked in my tight, shiny leggings.

'Oh' said youngest daughter, 'you've got your leather pants on'

I did a twirl expecting a compliment, such as wow hot momma etc.

'Like Ross in friends' was the slightly deflating comment, pissing all over my chips.

I spent the night making fart noises every time I moved on the chair and sweating my flaps off.

The pants have been hidden deep in the depths of my wardrobe until I forget why I never wear them and take them out for a spin again.

In another surprising move, husband and I joined a gym (it has a pool for me, I hate the gym) so I went swimming at 9am this morning, full of marvellous, sprightly keep fit intentions.

Alas, aqua aerobics was on, taking up two thirds of the pool. It was a well attended class with lots of eager ladies jumping up and down and hopping from side to side. This made the pool about as calm as a sea in a force ten gale to swim in.

Wave after wave crashed over me as my head valiantly bobbed and battled through the stormy waters to reach the end of the pool. After 20 lengths I gave up, utterly exhausted. I had, quite possibly, swallowed more water in my mouth and up my fanny than I had actually swam in.

I collapsed into the hot tub and promptly ingested, courtesy of a surprisingly positioned jet, yet more water straight up my foo foo.

Feeling thoroughly internally cleansed, I went to the changing room, which was now packed with the 900 ladies that had finished aqua aerobics, and, to my horror, promptly released the gallons of water from my insides thanks to the worlds loudest and most inappropriately timed fanny fart.

I think I'll give it a miss next week.

Wear The Shorts….
8th September 2021

Ah, a heatwave – lovely blue skies and sunshine plus unexpected hours after work in the garden. Bliss.

Except that I had just got excited about wearing leggings, jeans and tights again to cover my legs and baggy jumpers to cover everything else.

So, on Sunday, it was with some reluctance that I fished out my shorts again. Apart from holidays abroad, I can't remember the last time I wore shorts out in public in this country. I have always thought my legs, with their varicose veins and wobbly bits were far too unattractive to expose. My bum is saggy, not some lovely pert peach that hugs the seat of jeans or shorts in a sexy way. My arse just sort of hangs there, with a few random hairy bits. For as long as I can remember, I have considered wearing three quarter length pants as being as near to shorts as I can face.

And so, it was with a heavy heart full of self-loathing I went to put on my shorts. As I bent over husband wolf whistled. It suddenly occurred to me that he doesn't see an ancient saggy arse on flabby legs. He sees a curvy bum on shapely pins and fancies a bit of it.

Just as I don't notice any of his supposed flaws, to me he is gorgeous and very sexy, he looks at me and likes what he sees, so why can't I?

This was a revelation that, I think, has been a long time coming. All these years I have been overly critical of my weight and my imperfections but really, who gives a flying fuck except me?

So, I shaved off 3 bin bags worth of hairy legs and flaps, put drain buster down the plug hole and wore my shorts out to the shops! And nobody pointed and sniggered. Nobody said anything nasty and husband kept trying to have a sneaky leg feel in the car. I felt attractive and empowered. And really annoyed with myself that it has taken me until I am 50 to throw off the negative body image I have had for too long.

Our bodies may not be the perfect ones we see in magazines, but at least mine is real and not airbrushed. My body has fought off childhood illness with just a Dettol bath and a bottle of Lucozade, has carried two babies in quick succession, has country danced, maypole danced, disco danced, slow danced, drunken danced and belly danced, has run, walked, stretched, played hockey, netball, tennis and swam, and now it is a little bit older and a little bit knackered and at times it feels broken, frankly, but it is my body and I am proud of it.

I leak when I sneeze, I fart every time I get up from a chair, I will always have an armpit that grows hair quicker than the other, I couldn't hold a shit in if you paid me to, I'm exhausted by 9.30pm, I wake up with a nice set of whiskers and Mother Nature appears to think my minge hair needs to be 2 foot long with a few wispy bits growing out of my bum hole to balance things up, but I have learnt to love my body and it is about fecking time. I hope after reading this you will learn to love yourself too, because you are fricking fabulous.

Farting in the Frozen Food Aisle
Monday 25th October 2021

Well, I for one am glad to see the back of the full moon. This month my stomach bloated so much it needed its own postcode.

I even became a little bit attached to my enormous gut; it reminded me of being heavily pregnant and I was half wanting someone to ask me when the baby was due so that I could reply '20 years ago, you nosey bitch'. However, what goes up must, inevitably, come down and, alas, my stomach decided to deflate in the middle of Asda. Never have I longed so much for a screaming kid to distract from the violent eruption of noise blasting out of my bottom.

It all started in the frozen food aisle. I discovered, much to my surprise, that when I pressed my bloat against the side of the freezer to reach some burgers, I let out a massive fart. Startled almost as much as the man next to me, I quickly glared at him in mock horror for the benefit of anyone who had smelt but didn't know who had dealt, recoiled in horror from the burgers, stuck my nose in the air, and moved my trolly quickly over to the vegetables like I had suddenly turned vegan. Only for the same thing to happen again by the frozen peas.

I moved to the frozen potato section. By now bending over was an agony of wind and shame. I could only bend so far before the air squeezed out of the bloat and I blasted off. Looking like someone had shoved a metal pole up my jaxie, rendering me incapable of natural movement, I tried to stiffly semi-bend over the cabinet with my arms blindly flailing about trying to grab the items that I wanted.

Naturally, the one time this bloat eruption occurs in a supermarket there happens to be a fecking food shortage. So instead of overflowing freezers I was greeted with the scrapings at the bottom. I balanced precariously against the freezer, not quite able to reach the frozen chips, but scared of leaning over any more for fear of the inevitable.

The desire for chips overcame the desire to protect my dignity and so I bent over an extra inch, heard my arsehole let rip with gleeful abandon, grabbed my chips and wheeled off at top speed. Still farting. I found I was quite unable to stop.

Much like a deflating balloon whizzing round the room, I propelled my way round Asda non-stop farting. I decided not to bend down and get anything from the bottom shelves, it simply wasn't worth the risk.

All in all, it was quite a stressful shop, I had to keep wheeling my trolley away from different aisles so that people wouldn't suspect me, and, if I spied someone I had farted on before, I had to do an abrupt U turn and dive down another aisle.

I ended up buying crap that I don't need and we now have to live on chips, elderflower cordial, shoe polish and air fresheners, but I did at least leave the shop a dress size smaller.

Winter Vagina
16th November 2021

An article in the Daily Mail caught my eye yesterday. Do you suffer from winter vagina? Asked the headline, rather intrusively.

I have no idea, I said to myself. I better read on and have a look. Naturally, being the owner of a vagina about to head into the winter months, I was intrigued.

Did it mean your foo foo feels the cold and freezes shut from December to February?

Or did it mean you have a sudden urge to put tinsel and fairy lights in your growler and celebrate the season big time?

Alas, no.

In a nutshell winter vagina is basically having a dried-up fanny.

So, my winter stretches from January to fucking December and has lasted 5 years.

To add further insult to injury, there was a snide side column glowing with the joys of summer penis, where the male genitals spread out, stretch out and grow big and juicy during the hot summer sun, whilst I remain shrivelled and wrinkled like a reluctant tortoise.

The menopause is relentless, but you have to keep it real and you have to learn to laugh at the crap coming at you mentally, physically and hormonally.

That is why I am fed up of celebrities talking about how shit the menopause is while looking glossily groomed and glamorous and thin and bendy. I am especially sick of the tiny bikini poses and the washboard stomachs pictures. It almost feels like these celebrity women live in a different world where farts, pubic hair and rolls of fat simply don't exist. I am all for the sisterhood and I applaud you if you have managed to keep a fabulous figure, an even temperament and not lost your shagging mind, but keep it real for the sake of our sanity!

If I bend over without farting, I mark it on the calendar as a special occasion. Last week at keep fit/fat we did squats and I nearly passed out with the effort of keeping my pelvic floor inside me. When I exercise my face goes bright read, my hair frizzes up like I've been electrocuted and I sweat buckets. I grunt and mutter and curse under my breath. I clench my arse cheeks in for all I am worth in case I blast off, and I worry about pissing on the floor. I do not prance around all jolly and chirpy because it hurts, it is uncomfortable and I fucking hate it. But I do it to try and shift the two stone that menopause has dumped on me. I do it because I want to get fitter and I do it because, to a certain extent, there is now more pressure to look good in our 50's and not let ourselves go pleasantly to seed behind The Radio Times with a cup of tea and a custard cream. I compare myself to the celebs and find myself lacking. If the menopausal 50 plus celebs can pose up a storm in a teeny bikini with a washboard stomach, then who am I to hide my flab and poking out pubes behind my sarong, using the menopause as an excuse?

But the expectation to look fabulous is unreal and we need to remind ourselves to be more grounded.

So, celebs, show us what you really look like without the personal trainer, the cosmetic procedures, the make-up artists, the soft lighting, the stylist and the hairdresser. I applaud you for highlighting the menopause, but I want to see a sweaty, narky REAL woman pushing on through this shit show.

And if you suffer from winter vagina as well, so much the better. I'm off to get tinsel and baubles for my fandango and make the most of my seasonal suffering.

Fuck the Thong!
Monday November 29th 2021.

We are moving home soon, having decided after 11 happy years renting a cottage in the countryside, that the time is right to move into our own house. The new home is smaller and so there are things that must be got rid of. The last time we moved we were busy with work and so I left the packing to the removal guys, went off to work and came back at 6pm to a new home. Easy! But this time, in a rash and foolish move, husband and I have decided we can hire a van and do it ourselves. In another spectacularly rash and foolish move, we have decided that we would like to try and be in for Christmas.

We are therefore spending each evening going through our lifetime of belongings with a Keep! Sell! Charity! Throw! mentality that borders on the unhinged.

Last night it was the big chest of drawers in our bedroom. It consists of 8 drawers and husband had generously been allocated the top left drawer. All the others are mine. And they were bulging at the seams.

So, after 11 years of blissful ignorance, I was forced to sort out the hidden, forbidden depths of my underwear drawer. When we moved into our home, I was 39 years old. I am now fecking 50. This has been the home where middle age and the menopause have risen up and smacked me round the face.

Needless to say, the Sell! Charity! piles of my discarded and disgorged underwear drawers were non-existent. Drawer after drawer was emptied and I looked on in horror at how much underwear I actually had. It was fucking outrageous.

I decided to have new piles of Practical! Sexy! Tights! Socks! Fat days! Maybe one day! Never wearing the bastard cheese wire thing again! And No Chance!

The no chance pile grew ever bigger and I was astonished at how tiny my knickers used to be.

Progress was hindered by husband picking up my smalls from the no chance pile and asking why I didn't wear said item any more. I know love is blind, but if he couldn't see that the tiny scrap of lace he was dangling could now be anything other than a fucking chin strap then he needs urgent eyecare.

Finally, I had finished and was left with a pile of 'sexy' things in shagging size XL, fat day things, practical piss pad pants, woolly tights, socks and few maybe one day things. Feeling grumpy, I tried on one of my sexy XL nighties and do you know what? I looked pretty damn good. Before I could change my mind, I chucked all the teeny tiny pants away, facing up, at last, to the fact that a different woman is leaving the house to the one that arrived here 11 years ago.

And this woman can rock a pair of practical pants, had to shave her chin for the first time on Sunday because the bristle defeated the tweezers and doesn't need to wear a tiny thong to feel sexy. It was a small and long overdue adjustment, but I feel so much better for it

I'm not one for showing off my underwear in public, but I think this picture probably shows the before and after ravages that middle aged spread and menopause can inflict better than anything I can write, but you are still gorgeous and sexy and fabulous.

Rock those big pants ladies. You've got this. Fuck the thong!

Legs Bums and Tums
Monday 21st February 2022

A few days ago, in a moment of blind stupidity, I agreed to go to a legs, bums and tums class. In my deluded menopausal mind, I assumed this would be an aerobics style dance class with lots of middle aged, slightly wobbly ladies shaking their stuff and having a good boogie, all while trying to shed some lard.

Alas, when I opened the door, I did not see row upon row of comforting jelly bellies and smiling faces. No. My eyes looked despairingly at very fit, toned, slim people wearing tiny cropped vest tops and swishy hair. Even the men. And the hair was only swishing on their heads, not blowing in the breeze from armpits or growlers. I felt very out of my depth.

I pulled my extra-large snoopy T-shirt down to make sure I covered my camel hoof, always so prominent in lycra, and stood as close to the fan as was humanly possible. I took comfort in knowing I had surely to God walked into the wrong class.

Alarm bell 1: 'Turn the fans off' shouted the instructor, clearly a sadist.

Alarm bell 2: 'Anyone have any back problems or fitness issues?'

Alarm bell 3 'This is legs bums and tums' Oh Fuck, I was in the right place.

Alarm bell 4: 'But I run it as hardcore Pilates' Double fuck

Alarm bell 5: 'I do a 6-minute plank section in the middle' Fuck off.

I'd love to tell you that I sweated it out and emerged triumphant and 4 stone lighter, punching the air like Rocky. Instead, with as much dignity as I could muster, I stood up, walked to the front of the class, put my mat back and said, no thank you. To be fair, all the glossy, swishy, tiny vest people were really sweet and encouraging, but I knew I would be crap at the back of the class and, more to the point, I knew it wasn't right for me. I can never get my upper body to bend over my overflowing flab shelf and touching my toes is something I last achieved in 1996. Now I can only get halfway down my legs and that's with the aid of a massive fart. So, I walked out. Perhaps I should feel ashamed of myself, but feck it, knowing I had spared my body unimaginable pain and shame I felt 10ft tall.

Instead, I went on the bikes and cycled until my fanny was screaming.

On Saturday night, the husband and I had a housewarming party. I mentioned that I had recently acquired a device from Anne Summers and suddenly there was a stampede of ladies up the stairs and on my bed – 7 of us in all – each having our noses (thankfully only noses, and thankfully it was clean) tickled by the acquisition. The average age of us must be 52 for God's sake. It was one of those moments when you realise your friends are actually fucking feral after several gallons of prosecco. And that is, of course, why I love them so much. Naturally, the menfolk were too scared to come up and see what had become of their wives, but my husband will be thinking of seven ladies shrieking on his bed playing with one of Anne Summers finest for a very long time.

The night ended with a stunning impromptu performance by the ladies of Oops Upside Your Head which basically consisted of the back of the chain doing it fantastically out of time, as only the very pissed can, and Mrs C collapsed on top of me at the front, rendering both of us incapable of any movement. My flaps, still recovering from their workout on the cycle saddle – which was made from 100% freshly sharpened razor blades – bellowed in agony as my legs were forced to remain in a spread-eagled position for the entire length of the song. It almost made me nostalgic for legs, bums and tums.

Dear Menopause
28th March 2022

Dear menopause,

Why are you so cruel? Why do you have to take all my good bits away? My looks, figure and memory have all gone shit shaped.

My face is being pulled downwards, possibly by the weight of the beard that I grew overnight. I have jowls a bloodhound would take exception to. My face, unless I am smiling, defaults to abject misery or murderous fury. I no longer have an inoffensive, slightly pensive, neutral expression, I permanently look like someone has shit in my handbag.

I'm knackered from carrying an extra two stone around with me and fucked off from trying to shift it.

I don't sleep because my brain, which exists in a state of dormancy all day long, barely able to operate enough to complete a sentence or remind me what my kids are called, springs to life as soon as my head hits the pillow. Round and round my thoughts whirl, reminding me of all the cock ups I made during the day and taunting me with flashes of my former abilities.

And when I do, finally, mercifully fall asleep I am woken up in the small hours because I am on fire and melting thanks to the 4am flush.

I have to shave bits of me I didn't even know could grow hair – do I need a hairy arsehole? I managed quite well without one for 40 odd years but now, suddenly I have a furry bush full growing out of my crack. Yet, paradoxically, the hair on my head slowly thins and turns brittle and dull.

And, why dear menopause, do you wreak all of this havoc on me in the shadow of celebrities the same age who look a million fucking dollars with their glossy locks and their six packs and their shapely, tanned legs that do not look like corn beef or have big blue veins resembling the motorway network running up and down them. Celebs wear strappy little sandals and do not have a hairy yeti big toe or flankles.

Does the menopause not happen to women with money, or do they buy their way out of it?

I just don't want to know.

Dear menopause, you make me feel shit most of the time, but you have given me a palate to appreciate gin, a gob that I can't control and a wonderful, unstoppable urge to not give much of a crap about what people think. You have also given me empathy. I can empathise with those out there who feel stressed, anxious, bewildered, angry, narky, knackered and have a slightly damp gusset all at the same time. What special gifts you have bestowed on me.

Thanks for that

Sarah

Memory Lane
30th April 2022

Today I took my dog, Dennis, for a walk. I was halfway through when I realised I was walking down a lane very much like the one near where I grew up in West Oxfordshire. I used to walk our golden retriever down the lane when I was 15 or so and had no idea where life was taking me.

If I squinted, my golden lab, Dennis, could almost be our beloved old retriever. Under no circumstances could I be mistaken as my 15-year-old self, but it was suddenly easy to remember myself as I was; princess Di flicked hair, slender and fabulously carefree, feeling first love in all its cruel glory.

I wondered what my 15-year-old self would make of me today. She probably would've been horrified that I was no longer a size 10 and she might of been a little scornful that I'd let myself go.

I retaliated and told my 15-year-old self that at least I wasn't lying in bed at 8:20 on a sunny Saturday morning. But then I remembered that I had a Saturday job at 15 and my friend Robyn and I would be taken into Debenhams in Oxford by her mum.

I wondered what I would say to my 15-year-old self if I had the chance? Would I tell her that lovely, funny Robyn wouldn't make it to 40?

I'd tell her that her first love, will, in years to come, be nothing more than a rueful smile.

I'll tell her that boyfriends will come and go, but that she will have her heartbroken so badly every single piece of her will hurt. And it will teach her not to settle for second best.

I'll tell her that she thinks she will never want to fall in love again, but she will.

When you least expect it and when you least want it, because you are living a fantastic life in your flat with a good job, great social life, and your beautiful rescue dog, Joe.

Just when you are, for the first time, really enjoying being single and carefree, a man will walk into your office and that will be that.

One year and 15 days after your first date you will be married.

He literally will be your better half: kind and patient where you are rash and impatient, he is a gentleman, thoughtful and measured to your headstrong, he's a little bit shy and you are gob shite. He will always just be there.

He will hold you up when your beloved grandma dies and it will take all of your strength to put him back together when his father dies.

Would I tell younger Sarah that she has yet to experience the many months and months crying into a big fluffy towel when her period arrives because she so longs to have a baby?

She buries her face into the towel, heaving out big heart wrenching, grasping sobs from the depths of her soul because the towel muffles the sound. And because she loves her husband, she will dry her eyes and come out of the bathroom with a little smile, shake her head and say not this month.

And Joe the dog will whine and kiss away her salty tears.

She will sit in front of an expensive fertility consultant and be told that endometriosis has ravaged her so badly it's very unlikely that she will be able to conceive naturally, and her world will literally crumble. But the dreadful weight of trying to conceive, the crushing, suffocating, all-consuming pressure that leaves you a hollowed out version of yourself, will lift and you will give yourself time to adjust. Three months later, to everyone's astonishment you will be pregnant.

Another baby will follow 14 months later and you will have the time of your life raising two fabulous girls.

You will meet the friends of your lifetime along the way and getting older just happens as the world is measured by sports days, nativity plays and harvest festivals.

Through all this, your husband will be by your side, you will love him, laugh with him, and be infuriated by him. You will cry together when you have to let darling Joe go to sleep, and you will cry together again years later when his successor, chocolate lab Harry, king of the side eye, has to follow.

And I realise that this conversation to my 15-year-old self has actually turned into a bit of a love letter to my husband.

As I near the end of the lane, there is David waiting with the car to take me and Dennis home to save us walking all the way back uphill.

Young Sarah, life will have its fair share of ups and downs, but you will find a good man, and, feck me sideways, he will be worth the wait.

Dear Beloved

25th May 2022

A letter you may want to leave lying around somewhere...

Dear beloved significant other,

This is your menopausal partner speaking. I have found a rare moment of calm in between the storms that rage around my body and my brain to sit down and write a letter to you.

I know I am not the same woman you fell in love with. Physically I am bigger, OK fatter, I am obviously older and, alas, excessively hairier.

Mentally, I am a fucking fruit cake.

I have written this letter to try and help you understand what the hell is going on.

Facially – I know I have billy goat chin hair and jowls like a bloodhound. I know I look like a miserable cow most of the time. That is because I am. Wouldn't you be if your features were sliding down off your face thanks to gravity?

Mood swings - It might appear that, at times, I actively dislike you, but don't take it personally, I hate everybody and everything (except the dog) when in the rage zone. The truth is, I do love you very much but sometimes, from nowhere, uncontrollable anger boils up inside of me and explodes out like lava, just because you are chewing something loudly or breathing. I know it is unreasonable. But I do not care. So, when you see my eyeballs go red and my hairy nostrils flare, it is a good idea to remove yourself from close contact with me and ignore whatever spews out of my raging gob.

Do not try and argue back because that will make me cry.

Do not try to be nice to me because that will enrage me further.

Do not try and make sense of it – it is inexplicable.

Just pour me a glass of my favourite tipple and leave me to it.

It will soon be over.

Sex - bad luck. It is either feast or famine and even on a feast day you only have a three-minute window before I go off it again. And you don't get extra time to search for the tube of lube. But keep trying. I still fancy you, as long as you are not chewing or breathing too loudly.

Personal hygiene – I know I spend a fortune on lady pads, intimate wipes and adult nappies. Sorry about that. But the alternative is that I sit in a sea of piss every time I sneeze. The girl you met and married did not have a wheelie bin sized fanny with flaps down to her knees, and her pelvic floor worked like a charm. But shit happens and this is what you've ended up with. You push a satsuma out of your snake eye and see how much piss you can hold in afterwards.

Apologies, felt a bit of rage creeping in there for a moment.

Hot flushes – these are awful. I feel like I am being boiled alive. It is not helpful to suggest I look like I need to cool down, or to say that I look a little red, or ask me if I know I am sweating. Of course, I frigging know! It is cascading off me in buckets! Just get the fuck out of the way and get me a fan. And a Gin. With lots of ice.

Memory – You sometimes look concerned and perhaps occasionally think of taking me to a care home. Small wonder when I forget what I am saying whilst I am in the middle of shagging well saying it. I look and sound like an absolute knob most of the time. The old me was professional, articulate, organised and queen of multi-tasking. The new me can't remember what I walked in the room for. Unless it is the bedroom and that is because I remember that I will spend the entire bastard night tossing and turning thanks to insomnia. But don't book a guided tour of the care home just yet, memory loss and insomnia are all parts of the menopause – it's fecking great, isn't it?

I could go on, but I've forgotten what I was going to say.

Of course, all of this will hopefully, one day, pass and I might resemble my old self again. But they don't call it the change for nothing.

I am changing and I don't like it.

But love me anyway.

I am still in there under all this extra body hair. The fact that I can read this post and share it with you shows that there is life in the old girl yet. There are remedies out there and I have tried many, many things but I find laughter, talking about it and enjoying a glass of gin/vodka/wine/fizz to be the best tonic.

Now, ignore my moustache, give me a kiss and get your kit off, you've got three minutes.

For All the Women
24th June 2022

For all the women:

I know you feel down sometimes, I know you feel sad, lonely, confused invisible and tired. I know you sometimes feel as flat as a witch's tit, or as unwanted as a strap on in a nunnery.

I know this because I feel it too.

The menopause is hard, it takes our dignity, it takes our figures, and it takes our memory. We feel like we are slowly going mad. The menopause robs us of all these things and yet we get up every day and carry on regardless.

Regardless of feeling like shit most of the time, regardless of despairing that our jeans are tighter and regardless of the fact that every day we feel a little bit more of ourselves slipping away.

We clean, we cook, we wash, we mend, we work, we think, we solve, we are challenged, we are challenging, we love, we hope, we dream just the same as we did before but we carry this invisible burden inside of us. We are mourning the loss of our youth, we are mourning the loss of a glowing complexion, of supple skin, of a toned stomach, of shapely legs, of a face without fecking stubble, of joints that don't ache, of a memory that isn't foggy and dull, of the ability to shine and sparkle and be noticed.

Christ! We miss being even tempered and measured instead of being able to rage, scream, cry, laugh hysterically, insist we are fine, piss, fart and snot bubble all at the same fucking time.

We are shit scared that we are unattractive, going slowly round the pole and that we will be left alone.

At some point during the menopause, I think you fall out of love with yourself, you feel invisible and you feel worthless. All those plates you have been spinning for so many years - trying to balance being the best wife, the best mum, meal times, school runs, organising birthday's, parties, holidays, Christmas, being good at your job, running a home, and finding time to be fun, look good and be sexy - somewhere along the way you just let those plates stop spinning and fall to the floor without caring very much about it.

So, perhaps the biggest challenge we must overcome, is to learn to fall back in love with ourselves.

Not many of us can look in the mirror stark flap naked and honestly say we like what we see. Our eyes, diluted by unattainable perfection from the media, are drawn only to our flaws. I see way too much extra flab around my stomach, I see stumpy legs with varicose veins, I see mother nature doing her best to really piss me off.

I am not kind to myself; I do not look and see a 50-year-old woman whose body has produced two beautiful children, and whose stomach has enjoyed many lovely long lunches and fabulous parties. I criticise and fault find because I do not look like a bastard barbie doll.

So, for all the women out there having a crappy day; I know how you feel because I feel it too. I will say to you what I need to say to myself: you are beautiful, you are worthy of the love that comes your way, you deserve to feel good. You may not be shining or sparkling today but perhaps you will tomorrow.

You are fucking glorious.

A different shaped body just needs different sized clothes but can still be knock out sexy, a crop of chin hair that grows so fast it needs harvesting every morning can be plucked or waxed or shaved. A bit of make-up goes a long way. A glass of gin goes even further.

For all the women: you are so worth the effort and don't ever doubt otherwise.

The Cycle of Shit
Tuesday 5th July 2022

As I have been bounced along through middle age, I have come to appreciate that my menopause journey has a clear monthly cycle. Naturally, it is a cycle of solid gold shit but it does have definite stages.

Week one: All aboard for stress, anxiety, insomnia, massive belly overhang where nothing fucking fits, misery, despair, exhausted and generally pissed off. Fanny as dry as a drought in the Sahara. Cry at Shirley Valentine.

Week two: Anger surges through my veins like lava and simmers waiting for an opportunity to erupt, usually over a missing pan lid or a spoon put the wrong way up in the dishwasher, my husband is deliberately snoring to annoy the fuck out of me and everyone is a complete fucking arse. Tempted to book flights to Greece and work in Costa's Taverna. Chips and egg anyone?

Week three: Experience the great hair growth and have to shave face – FACE! – legs, bum, growler, armpits, every shagging day. This is also the week I will produce the world's longest grey eyebrow hair and the 12-inch tucked away and hitherto invisible chin hair. Both will uncurl and unfurl in a very public place, like a queue, poking the neck of the person in front of me. Mood improves as quickly as hair grows, and, after a shave, I realise I am not that bad. Drop into Nympho mode. Husband likes this week.

Week four: Stomach finally deflates and I can see my granny fanny in all it's glory. Horrible old lady grey hair straggles back at me and is removed with all haste. This is also the week my muff gets hungry and chews up toilet roll with indecent haste, which I forget to check because I have severe brain fog, so muff spits out lumps of bog roll in the swimming pool changing room.

I am currently on week four, so my apologies in advance to the ladies of Telford Aqua Fat if you find strange clumps of loo roll dotted around the changing room this week.

Eat it

Sunday 24th July 2022

Yesterday I had to buy some fat sucky in pants and was served by a 15-year-old boy in M & S. He was mortified. I was horrified, squirming with shame watching a teenage boy handle my giant marquee pants with extreme distaste. And one of them was a thong approximately 8 ft wide. He looked a bit sick at that point. Even I was wincing as he got swallowed by a pair whilst looking for the label. When he emerged, he was sweating. I've probably put him off women for life.

I blame the menopause for my weight gain. Let's face it, I blame it for fecking everything. But, to be fair, since being menopausal I have noticed slight glitches to my diet.

For example, if I am eating a tub of Ben & Jerry's ice cream, otherwise known as crack, I don't just have a couple of slurps. Oh no. I eat halfway down the tub and then apply the fabulous logic that I had better eat the rest of the shagging thing to get rid of it so that it is gone.

Ditto with a chocolate bar. I'm at it like a truffle pig complete with grunts and snorts. I think my bum wiggles a bit in excitement too. In it all goes.

My brain thinks it makes perfect sense to snaffle the lot because then I can't eat it.

My brain refuses to process the fact that I already have eaten it.

Interestingly, I do not apply this thought process to leafy salad or fresh fruit or shitty cardboard Ryvita.

The menopause is sly, filling my brain with hormonal cravings for ice cream and chocolate whilst ensuring any desire to exercise is chemically removed via the exodus of testosterone. Off go all the energetic little hormones and in come the lazy fat bastard hormones. And the delusional hormones that make you believe eating a whole tub of ice cream is actually a good thing.

Because then you can't eat it.

The menopause might be shit, but you can't argue with its logic.

Mr X-rated
2nd August 2022

A great friend of ours, whom I shall call Mr X, has recently been very ill and we have all been deeply concerned about him. Quite simply he is the life and soul of any party and I cannot image a life without him in it. Mr X recently received the fabulous and hugely relieving news that he is now better, and he decided to throw a party to celebrate.

Mr X makes a very mean punch which tastes completely harmless but results in you losing three days and waking up on Snowdonia with your knickers on your head. I was wise to the punch and only had two glasses and then dived into the Prosecco. Husband foolishly had several pints of the stuff and went sweaty, twirly and waxy faced. His best friend kindly fortified him with whiskey.

We danced and drank and celebrated life.

All in all, it was a marvellous night

However, when Salt n Pepa come on and you screech Get Up On This! Whilst pointing to your own aging groin in front of your friend's horrified 22-year-old son, you know you are losing the war with drink.

We left and zig-zagged home at around 2am.

It is fair to say we live in OAP Ville and to see folk out and about on our street at that time of the morning usually means somebody has died.

So, we were astonished to see a group of young people coming towards us as we stumbled home. Husband and I stood by to let them past and I said 'ooh look a coach party' and then cracked up at my hilarity. One of the coach party said 'hello mother' and I had the appalling realisation that neither of us had recognised our own child. In our defence it was dark, we are old, we didn't have our glasses on. And we were spectacularly shit faced

To make amends, yesterday I decided to print out a picture of my offspring, taken at her graduation, to put on a wall at home. I duly took my phone to the chemist and plugged it in.

As usual there was a crowd of people in there, the chemist is tiny and wherever you stand your business can be seen and overheard. There was genuine shock that I didn't head straight to the piss pad aisle. I nodded and smiled to everyone and said I was printing off my daughter's graduation pictures, and yes, it was a marvellous day and yes, I was very proud.

I selected the most recent 25 photographs and up they flashed in all their glory. The chemist was hushed into appalled silence as pictures of Mr X's willy were beamed on the screen. The cheeky bastard, under the influence of his own lethal punch, had pinched my phone and managed several charming self-portraits of his penis. Alas, with no face attached to the images, all the oldies thought it was my husband winking at them. A few of them winked back at me for good measure.

The circle of life at its finest: Mr X gets better and I die of shame.

Big Daddy
Wednesday August 31st 2022

I was just pondering ordering a pair of shorts to wear in the autumn and winter months, obviously with million denier tights and boots. Instead, and rather disappointingly, I ordered my traditional boot cut black trousers with a slightly elasticated waist.

The 25-year-old me was screaming 'order the fucking shorts!' but the 25-year-old me can shag off because she was half the size and her thighs didn't create friction burn sparks that would be a fire hazard.

In fact, when I was 25, I did not have the confidence to wear a fabulous pair of shorts with tights and boots. I really didn't appreciate how good my figure was, and, now that I have occasional flares of confidence, I find I am limited by my own restrictions as to what I think is appropriate for a curvy woman to wear. In shorts I picture myself looking like I'm morphing between Giant Haystacks and Big Daddy.

And yet, I see women bigger than me looking amazing and not giving a shit. I want some of that.

My friend told me off recently for being too negative about myself on this page. But I think a lot of us are hard on ourselves and arm ourselves with baggy clothes and a sense of humour to hide the inner horror we feel at watching ourselves turn into hairy old women.

All aboard for anger, tearfulness, insomnia, hot sweats, lethargy, flatulence, incontinence, mild alcoholism, memory loss, flab bulges popping out, pubes falling out, one eyebrow hair with abnormal growth, impossible to pluck chin bristles and hairy feet.

If you cannot hide away whilst all this happens, or take HRT, then it takes work to look good: much shaving, plucking, waxing, dyeing, squeezing, pushing, stuffing, shoving etc, plus make up and flattering clothes. Then you have to change clothes at least 5 times before going out because you don't feel nice, which makes you sweaty and cross and pissed off before you even set foot outside.

The menopause makes us feel fat and ugly and then saps our energy so much we can't be bothered to wrestle with a pair of Spanx and a stubborn roll of flab, so we stick to the same uniform of elasticated waists and think the world should count itself lucky we have removed our moustache. On days like this my favourite word is Fuck.

But today, I have decided to make the effort and, after reading this back, I have gone and ordered the shorts.

They probably won't fit and I'll look like a twat.

But it is a start.

A positive new me.

With a colossal camel's toe.

Vabbing
7th September 2022

I've just read about 'Vabbing' in the Daily Mail.

Vabbing, in case you are completely in the dark - which is where I was 30 minutes ago, and what a lovely place that was - is where women dab or rub a bit of what I can only call vagina juice onto their whereabouts instead of perfume.

The thought being that your intimate scent will make you wildly irresistible to all who catch a whiff. Something to do with pheromones.

I don't know if I even still have any pheromones, perhaps there is a single weary pheromone floating around inside me, shrivelled and knackered.

I don't think it will smell very nice.

I read this article about Vabbing out to the guys in the office, one of whom is my husband. they both looked revolted, none more so than husband who, rather unflatteringly for my vag juice, went green and looked like he wanted to puke.

Maybe this Vabbing lark is designed for non-menopausal women. Perhaps you can only vab if you have a pelvic floor that actually works and don't have elephant ear fanny flaps hanging halfway down your leg.

I'm not sure Eau de fish market with top notes of piss is going to attract anything other than flies, so I'll sit this one out.

Dear me
September 18th 2022

We often think of what we would write and tell our younger self, if only we had the chance.

I've done it here on this blog - things I would say to the 15-year-old Sarah with the benefit that only hindsight and life experience through age can bring.

But now, out of nowhere and for reasons I cannot quite fathom, I am going to imagine myself as a crusty, musty old bird many years from now, and think what my future self would say to me today, given the chance.

Dear middle aged Sarah,

You don't know it and you certainly don't feel it, but you are in the prime of your life at the moment. Yes, your body is falling apart and everything aches like shit (yes, dear, the future you still swears like a trucker) but it all still works. Your brain might fog up every now and then but it is sharp and quick at other times. Use it more.

One day you will look around and see that winter has set in. In your bones and in your life. The sand is running far too fast through the timer. All these things you bother about now will be irrelevant in the future and not worth the frown lines.

Be kinder to yourself.

Sleep doesn't come easy to you now, but one day soon you will sleep far too soundly and be surprised to wake up at all. So don't stress about insomnia, don't worry about material things, one day all these niggles will be a distant memory.

You have put on weight. So what? Stop squeezing into clothes that are too small and hating yourself for it. Buy bigger clothes, go brighter, bolder. Life is too short to be a wallflower.

Travel. See the world. You are a long time dead my girl. So don't leave it until your bones ache so much the mere act of going down the local Co-op is the equivalent of an expedition to Everest. Get out there and do it now, while you can. One day you will struggle to get around. That creaky sound and pain in your knee will worsen over time and you will need a walking stick. Enjoy walking tall and moving freely.

Don't wait until your hands are wrinkled and gnarled with liver spots and age, use them now to write that book, paint that picture, play that instrument.

Eat well, enjoy that drink and don't compare yourself to others. You are enough. You don't need or want to starve yourself thinner. Trust me, your future self thinks your current body is knockout. Your boobs are still in roughly the right place and your arse isn't yet at the back of your knees. So shimmy on and strut your stuff - embrace those curves, believe you are gorgeous.

Cherish your family and your friends, the future you misses these times and longs to see much loved faces again.

The future you is reading this in tears thinking of times when you could have and should have done more and said more with the people you love the most.

Don't take love for granted.

Don't take life for granted.

Time marches on and it's wasted on the young.

And you are still young.

Celebrate life, laugh more, do more, be more.

This is your time if only you knew it.

And I'm not crusty or musty, thank you very fecking much!

With love and wisdom,

Old lady Sarah x

The Early Morning Call
Thursday 22nd September 2022

A sad and rather surprising fact I have learnt about getting older is that my husband and I now spend more time farting at each other first thing in the morning than we do actually talking.

I woke myself up this morning, arse flapping like elephant ears, with a very loud blow off. It woke my husband up as well as me. He responded with one of his own, but as this was on the toilet, I am not allowed to include it or write about it because the toilet is a sacred and safe space for bottoms.

There followed puff ping pong; back and forth our bottoms blew at each other in turn. It wasn't deliberate, I just don't think either of us either know we are doing it or, in my case, can actually help it.

Down I bent to retrieve yesterday's knickers from the floor and out came a fart.

Up I stood as quickly possible and out came another banger. Off I staggered to the wash basket releasing a volley of farts along the way. Husband reciprocated, although he will deny this. This went on for a few minutes before either of us uttered a word.

And then we just starting chatting as if this morning's windy waffling was just a normal part of everyday life that has slid into our world without us batting so much as an arsehole. When, and more importantly, why did this happen?

When we first got together, I wouldn't fart in front of my husband if you paid me to. My stomach used to ache from holding one in and I'd sneak off to his bathroom and blow off against his towels to muffle the sound. Husband kept encouraging me to just relax and release, but I refused. I come from a long line of loud and proud flatulence kings (hello, Dad) so I knew what was coming and loved him enough to spare him. Also, I wasn't sure if he'd stick around.

But, the minute we got engaged I felt like a weight had been lifted. So, I let go, blew myself around the room and it has been that way ever since.

I was just a bit surprised to realise how much time first thing of a morning is taken up just blowing off and why we hadn't noticed it before. I promise, dear husband, to make more effort to actually speak in the mornings. I will converse with you and say good morning/how did you sleep/no chance until I've had a cup of tea/I don't care if it is bigger in the mornings etc before I consciously let rip.

The unconscious fart is beyond my control, but, going forwards, I will try to say 'excuse me' instead of 'I bet you can't beat that!'

Welcome to Middle Age
26th September 2022

Welcome to middle age, life looks good, maybe a bit of money in the bank, small or no mortgage, couple time, travel time.

I was quite excited for this time in our lives: that time when the kids learn to drive and have independence, leave home to go to university or just generally spread their wings away from home a bit more. After the chaos and battle ground from toddler tantrums to teenage arguments and all the bits in-between; getting them up for school, finding out it is PE and the kit is mouldering in the bottom of a bag somewhere, or worse, just as you are leaving the house being told it is shagging cookery class, performances, assembly's, PTA meetings, parent's evenings, washing, ironing, ferrying around. Endless one-sided conversations where I would try to find out what my offspring had been doing all day:

'How was school?'

'Boring'

'What did you do?'

'Nothing'.

It has been a privilege and a pain all at the same time.

So, slightly bedraggled from raising two children, and overwhelmed with pride that they had both made it to university, I sat back and waited for smug middle age to wash over me. I had time to do my hair and make-up of a morning, time to go shopping for nice new things, time to do yoga, belly dancing, the gym. Time to be sexy and glamorous, flirty and fun.

Alas, the only thing that washed over me was a hot flush.

Just as I have reached the time in my life where I can put me first, I find that I can't be arsed to do anything.

May becomes October in the blink of an eye and the biggest achievements I have managed are finding a decent box set to watch and not eating all the Minstrels in a family pack.

I haven't gone to the gym, I haven't done yoga or belly danced.

I have phases where I will get a surge of energy, will remember that I am a woman with needs, that this is supposed to be my time and I will undertake a massive grooming effort to go from Wildebeest to sylph but unplugging the drain and removing bin bags of body hair is a bit of a passion killer, to say the least.

Asking where the KY Jelly is just sets me alight with lust.

Where have I gone? Who is this lethargic husk in my place?

My dress size has grown bigger as my brain gets smaller.

The 'one day it will fit' pile of clothes is now larger than my actual wardrobe.

My sexy knicker drawer has welded itself shut through lack of use.

I like Countryfile.

I joined the National Trust.

I like Home and Garden magazine.

I almost watched Antiques Roadshow.

My temper flares and flashes and then fritters away in a cloud of anxiety and apathy.

I can spend hours plucking my chin.

It really pisses me off when people do not respect my sofa cushion placement.

I cry, I shout, I snap, I swear, I despair, I am happy, I am sad, I am angry I am numb. All at the same fucking time.

It is exhausting and yet I lie awake night after night trying to turn my brain off.

Whose bright idea was it to have the menopause crash land just as the kids were of an age to leave?

I did try to make the effort on Saturday night, applied makeup and felt fabulous.

I conversed in a highly intelligent and brilliant fashion, asking a musician if he played the trampoline instead of tambourine.

My husband asked if I was hot because my cheeks were perspiring.

It was highlighter….

I Spy
12th October 2022

Recently, my husband and I went to sell a car and got offered a fair price from a trader. We rocked up to our appointment but the little portacabin office looked shut.

Having had a journey of an hour to get to our destination and having unwisely drunk several cups of tea prior to leaving the house, I was bursting for a wee and was frankly more excited about visiting their toilet than I was about getting some £££ for the vehicle.

The office being closed sent a wave of panic through me and husband was made to go out of the car and try the door.

Definitely closed.

We sat for 10 minutes, well he sat and I fidgeted like a toddler, holding onto my growler. Husband got up and wandered around the site. No sign of anybody. I couldn't move and check it out myself, so urgent was the need to piddle.

Eventually, about 30 seconds later, my bladder went hysterical with the need to offload 14 gallons of tea and pee so I gingerly got out of the car like a 97 year old, no sudden movements less the stop tap gets disturbed, scratched around for a suitable hiding place behind the car, and prepared to slide my jeans and pants down and open the hatch.

I instructed husband to use my jacket as a shield as there was quite a busy road nearby and my flaps could be seen beneath our vehicle, should anyone feel inclined to look over our way.

Husband held the jacket up around my face.

'Lower!' I hissed as I pissed.

The blessed relief I felt was spoilt only by the fact that my wee was so ferocious I was unable to stop splash back on my lovely boots and had to watch helplessly as the unstoppable and never-ending pee left its mark on my tan suede.

We were very close to the ringway for Birmingham airport and a plane load of passengers had a pleasant start to their holiday watching me wee as their plane flew right over us on its ascent.

Husband wondered if I would be finished by the time they returned from holiday.

Finally, the tank was empty, I washed my boots down with water in a vain effort to disguise the fact that they were now soggy with piss, straightened up and we called the car dealer to find out where they were.

'There is a gate to the left of where your car is parked'

Came the worrying reply.

'We were just about come and get you'

Horror thrilled every nerve of my body as I realised it was not only a plane load of holiday makers who had borne witness to the indignities of my 10-minute wee, the pissing on my lovely boots and my futile attempts to be dignified and wash the evidence away while my bare arse waved about in the air.

Yes, my husband had merely man-looked when checking to see where the dealer was and hadn't noticed the big fuck off gate next to the portacabin, which led straight to a lovely shiny new office, open and welcoming, complete with toilet. And CCTV.

My Name Is Sarah
6th October 2022

Since I started this blog there are now so many new followers, I thought it might be a good idea to introduce myself to you all.

My name is Sarah. I began this blog back in 2018 when I started to notice that my toes were hairy, my hip ached and I was moody all the time.

Peri-menopause arrived and dumped on me. I soon had bloating, insomnia and a burning desire to call everyone a knob head.

At the time there was no real celebrity endorsement of the menopause. It wasn't out there. Everyone my age on TV looked thin and glossy and normal. They still do, to be fair. I don't like them.

I felt and looked like Les Dawson's Cissy and Ada. There had to be some humour in this madness and so that's what I have tried to do on this page.

I'm thrilled that more and more people are opening up about the menopause, but I can only tell you about my journey.

I swear a lot.

I sweat a lot.

I'm slightly overweight and can't be arsed to do shag all about it, except moan.

I feel anxious and itchy.

I ache all over first thing in the morning.

I'm wide awake every single night.

Most people get on my tits.

But I like having a giggle and I believe talking about the changes we experience is hugely helpful.

Did I think I would ever need to pluck my nipples?

Quite honestly, no.

Shave my toes?

Never.

Shave the top of my fecking feet, for God's sake?

Absolutely not!

Did I think I would have to wear a pad every day because wee seeps out?

Not at all.

Did I ever think there would come a time when I would feel stubble on my chin and utter the words 'not too bushy, I'll leave it another day?'

Nope.

Would I ever have looked in the mirror, seen a nice little clump of nostril hair and thought, sod it, I'll pluck it tomorrow?

Not a chance.

All these things would've horrified me not too long ago, but now it's just part of a normal day.

I often think I'd like to go out for a run or go to the gym but then I remember that I hate all that shite, park my bum on the sofa and eat a Twix.

I feel tired, fucked off and can fart the national anthem most days.

But I am still me, under these layers of horror, stress, shame and self-blame, I am in there somewhere fighting the good fight.

We are all still in there somewhere. We might be a bit bigger, hairier and whiff a bit. We might be narky, moody, hysterical, dead eyed, tearful, horny, irritable, irrational beings, but we are soft and squishy inside and riding a roller coaster that none of us wanted to get on.

So, this is me, 51 years old, married mum of two, chocolate loving, crisp eating, gin drinking me.

Brain Fog
11th October 2022

Brain fog.

One minute you are a successful, capable woman. You can run a household, raise a family and excel at your job. You can organise, arrange and multi task. You can think ahead, plan ahead and, in a calm efficient manner, can deal effectively with all life's little dramas. You can keep a shopping list in your head, plan a night out and book a holiday all at the same time. You can walk the dogs, go to yoga and do an Aldi big shop all in the same morning. You are fucking marvellous.

And then, you wake one morning and it is as if your soul has seeped into the mattress and left a husk that looks like you but has the ability to do shag all. Your brain is full of cotton wool. The answers are in there somewhere but it takes so long to climb through the fog that by the time you shout 'Mary Berry! Yes! I knew it!' in triumph, the conversation has already moved onto someone else who sounds vaguely familiar and was in something you are sure you used to watch if only you could remember what it was called.

Completing a sentence is beyond you, halfway through speaking you are blankly mouthing nothingness like a goldfish blowing bubbles. That marvellous, interesting point you had articulated in your brain, ready to come confidently out, sounding intelligent and fabulous has just vanished into thin air. Mid way through fecking saying it. You couldn't look more stupid if you tried to.

And that is the cruelty of brain fog, for whilst it is easy to forget what you were going to say, you are unable to forget that you were actually going to say something. There follows confusion as to what the hell is happening, shock that the words have dried up, horror that you cannot remember what on earth you were saying, fear that you have early onset dementia, anger that your brain has shit on you and resignation that you will no doubt recall the conversation at 3.04 AM.

So, if you work or live with a peri/menopausal woman, please print this out and refer to it next time you see a woman looking panicked because she has stopped speaking mid-sentence. She maybe muttering the words 'Bastard menopause, for feck's sake, bollocks not again' to herself and looking quite mad. I am here to tell you that the poor cow is not going round the bend she has been swallowed by the brain fog. Give her a break and make her a brew. Or pour her a gin if it is the afternoon. Feck it! Pour her a gin is it's after 7am. She deserves it.

The Cure All
Thursday 13th October 2022

The other night/early morning at 2.47 am, I was, as usual, wide awake and wondering why I couldn't sleep, when I rolled over onto my ancient old lady crumbling right hip and, for a few minutes, just watched my husband sleeping peacefully next to me.

There he was, sleeping deeply, breathing calmly in and out, not a care in the fecking world.

Marriage is all about sharing experiences, so I woke my husband up.

'Why am I awake?' came the baffled response.

'Now you know what it is like to be a menopausal woman' I said, helpfully.

'I've got a cure for that' was the unexpected reply.

He looked at his lad and looked at my mouth.

Ever hopeful.

Yes, ladies and gentlemen, according to my husband, the cure all really is a miracle and can actually cure the menopause. It must be swallowed a minimum of once a day every day for a year before you will see any effects, and then every day after that just to be on the safe side.

If my fecking leg fell off a well administered dose of the cure all would make a new one grow back.

If I would only take the recommended intake of at least 3 doses a day, husband says I would be happy and sailing through menopause right now without a care in the world.

Alas for husband, I would rather suffer the menopause and so he got the 3am knock back and I started to regret waking him up in the first place.

'Suck it to sleep?' Came a hopeful voice out of the darkness.

'No thank you'

'Stroke it sleep?'

'No'

Within seconds he was asleep again, dreaming his happy dreams and I was left admiring the fact that he can be woken up in the middle of the night, instantly be horny, talk bollocks, try it on, get the knock back and be back asleep again all within 5 minutes.

Men really are from a different planet.

She Was Fabulous
Wednesday 16th November 2022

Back in the mists of time, after a day at work I would often meet up with colleagues or friends for a drink, or go to the cinema, out for a meal or even pop to the gym. We would go into Manchester and hit the bars and clubs. When I got together with my husband, I would finish work and drive to his house, or he would come to mine. We used to be all over each other like a rash. We would also meet up with friends, go into town and just be out there living life. Energy. I had energy. And motivation.

Somewhere, somehow, I have morphed into a woman who now puts the key in the door, and, with a sigh of relief that I don't have to go out, aches and creaks her way upstairs, throws her pyjamas on, aches and creaks her way downstairs, puts the kettle on, lights the fire and sits her hairy arse on the sofa. I move to put the dinner on and let the dog out. I move to get chocolate out of the fridge. I move to go to the loo, clutching my hip which feels like it should be on a 98-year-old woman, not someone of 51. I move to ache and creak back up the stairs at 10 pm to go to bed.

Where the fuck have I gone?

Who is this old bat that looks like a bigger version of me, sounds like me but feels so old?

I'm looking forward to planting my bulbs this weekend. I want to go and look at sheds. Who am I?

I should add here that husband also gets in his PJ's, or lounge wear as he prefers to say, the minute he gets in, perhaps apathy is catching. The difference is that at 6am every morning, he is off and out to the gym whereas at 6am every morning I roll over, realise he has gone, let out a massive fart and stretch myself, starfish like, across the bed and go back to sleep. Fuck getting up at that time. Apart from walking the dog, this shuffling movement around the bed is my only form of exercise.

I know the menopause is to blame, but knowing that and being bothered to do something about it are two different things. And there is the issue laid bare. The menopause robs you of the inclination or motivation to fight your way out of it. Fair play if you can jump up and exercise, eat right, drink smoothies and be glossy and fabulous, but I feel weak. I want to eat shit and drink vodka. There are bumps in this journey and I have slumps, but there are also highs. Despite feeling like a dead sloth most of the time I also have unexpected confidence and have learnt to try and laugh at this madness. I talk to my husband and I talk to my friends. It keeps me just this side of sane.

I still mourn the person I was before mood swings, insomnia, itchy skin, chin stubble, hot flushes, incontinence, brain fog and fat thighs took hold. The person who could have an intelligent conversation and get the end without forgetting what she was saying. The person who could have spontaneous sex without scrabbling around for the lube because her fandango has run dry. The person who was normal. But that glorious creature was just a phase in my life, like being a toddler and a teenager. It is hard to let her go because she was fabulous and she just didn't appreciate how fabulous she was until she morphed into me. But this new me is OK. She is coping, she is finding new clothes to wear that are flattering instead of fattening. She slaps her make up on and makes the best of herself. In short, she is keeping her head above water. Mostly because if her moustache gets wet it will drag her under.

It is your journey so do whatever you need to do to get through it. Even if you find yourself doing absolutely fuck all.

Facial Versus The Fart
Thursday 24th November

I was having a scroll through Facebook the other day at some of the other menopause sites. They are quite lively and chirpy with multiple daily posts, catchy sayings and funny memes. It's all very nice.

Alas, I'm not finding the menopause a very chipper place to be – it is full of grey pubic hair, memory loss and piss pads. It is all a bit shit. I try to tell it like it is, I don't post every day because sometimes I can't be arsed to pick my dirty pants up off the floor, never mind sit and type a story from the heart.

When I write these blogs, I imagine I am sitting down with my friends and just letting it all out. I let out the shock and horror of what is happening to us, tell you how I try to cope and what symptoms I am experiencing. I let out most of my inner thoughts, I unleash my anger, and I try to find some humour as I watch myself turn into one of the ancient whiskery, half mad women of my childhood. My Christ, no wonder they swilled ginger wine and sherry down their necks. Imagine going through all of this without a support group, or without being able to say Fuck a lot.

Fuck that.

Yesterday I went for a facial, a surprise from my husband who was probably worried that his wife had turned into ZZ top. It was a lovely surprise, but because it was a surprise, I didn't have advance notice. All I could think was Shite! I haven't plucked my chin.

And, indeed, I hadn't plucked the fucker for a good few days. It had gone from angry, spikey bristle to a soft, light down. Much like a teenage boy sporting a wispy bit of fluff on his chin, my little beard fluttered and lifted in the breeze every now and then. From time to time, I found myself twirling it round my fingers.

Naturally I had mere slip of a girl doing the facial who undoubtedly had less hair on her fanny than I had on my chin.

I soon as I lay down, I wanted to fart. It's like a reflex. I prayed for her to leave the room in order to release. She didn't. I couldn't risk sneaking one out whilst she was there because, just lately, I have been very loud indeed. It is like a new string to my menopause bow. Also, there was a possibility I would've levitated off the bed with the blast, which would be startling for both of us, so I kept hold of it and tried not to relax too much.

I don't know if you've ever tried to not relax whilst having a facial. It's almost painful and made for some very strange expressions. I'm sure the therapist thought I was having an orgasm. Or a stroke.

My lady gave me a good scouring, as if trying to scrub away the wrinkles, and applied many expensive lotions and potions, presumably in a bid to make me want to buy the miracle products at the end of the session. She slapped quite a lot of oil around the chin area, as if trying to slick the hair down. It speaks volumes that the poor girl turned the lights down nice and low before showing me the results in the mirror. She would've been better turning the fucking light off. My beard was freshly oiled and my skin looked glowing but I think that was from the effort of holding in my huge fart.

I lied and said I looked fabulous, thank you very much but I would stick with my Aldi face cream after all. She left, I cocked a leg and blew off, then went to Tesco to buy some booze. I had just about reconciled myself to being a whiskery old woman pissed up on Stones ginger wine when, at some considerable cost, I suddenly and erratically swung the other way and ordered a permanent hair removal device from Amazon.

I'll let you know how it goes; I intend to use it everywhere. I almost feel sorry for it.

Monkey Nuts
Monday 19th December 2022

Last Friday was our works Christmas do. We are only a small team so no need to bother with airs and graces and awkward pauses. Because we all work in the same office, we all know rather a lot about each other and everyone knows everything about me, thanks mostly to my big mouth and this page which is reluctantly followed by one of my colleagues.

My husband and I started off by picking up our colleague and, naturally had to have a drink and some nibbles at her house first. I was wearing quite a low-cut top. Rather than the sexy hint of cleavage look I was hoping to achieve (my figure has gone to shit; boobs are all I have) I caught sight of myself and was, alas, reminded of a builder's bum crack. Complete with hair.

I knocked a drink back to get over the disappointment of having a bum crack rack, and ate a few monkey nuts.

Whenever I go out for a meal, I manage to drop mouthfuls of food on myself. In fact, to be truthful, this generally happens whenever I eat, wherever I am. I might as well throw a forkful of food on myself and be done with it. So, it came as no great surprise when some monkey nuts found their way down the crack rack. I fished about for a minute until I remembered that I was in somebody else's home and shoving a hand down my top to rummage for half a nut isn't really the polite thing to do.

Onwards to the pub where we met up with the rest of our gang. I ordered a truck load of booze on the work account and, because we had a 3 hour wait until our curry, I sensibly got some snacks. Crisps and peanuts filled the table. We drank and giggled and ate our snacks. I became vaguely aware that it had been an age since I had been to the loo. I then became very aware that I had drunk several pints. Instantly, my bladder screamed at me to empty it with all haste. I stood up and staggered as quickly as I could to the ladies.

I burst into trap one. Alas, alas I had forgotten that not only was I wearing my giant fat pants, obviously lined with a pad, I also had an all-in-one body on, complete with under carriage poppers.

In case it has been, like myself, many years since you were foolish enough to wear an all in one on a boozy night out, allow me refresh your memory: Firstly, if you have a large tummy, it is quite hard to achieve the right stance needed to under the poppers. You have to spread your legs and do a semi downward dog manoeuvre to be able to reach them. Then you have to fumble around for a few minutes trying to locate the poppers which have been half eaten by your greedy foo foo. You might start to do the I need a wee wee jiggle which makes locating the poppers even more difficult. Finally, you rip the poppers open in triumph and yank out several tuffs of pubic hair in the process. You are left with your saddle bag flaps flopping out of their confinement, either side of the wretched garment flailing around and several clumps of growler hair wafting to the floor.

Anyway, back to my predicament. I was eye wateringly desperate for a pee. Now! Screamed my bladder. Not yet, don't piss yet, hold it in, no, just one more second, please don't wee yet I replied to myself, unfortunately out loud. Finally, and barely in time, the poppers were released along with a monkey nut, three peanuts and a crisp all of which tumbled gleefully out and scattered under the cubicle sides. I then had to squeeze the fat pants down before slumping on the loo with a sigh of relief and a fart. At this point I heard a sniff of horror from trap two.

Yes. There had been somebody in the stall right next to me the whole time. Not only had they heard me charmingly trying to talk myself out of pissing my pants, they had faced an avalanche of snacks courtesy of my gusset larder and heard me let rip. Not my finest hour. Luckily, I was spared the shame of facing them due to the fact that I had to have a 20-minute pee. After that all I could do was drink and repeat the process several more times.

So, please, if you are heading off out this festive season, don't risk your dignity. Stick with the massive incontinence pants girls. Looking like Donald duck from the waist down has got to be better than bar snacks falling out of you.

The Shit Sea
19th Jan 2023

One day, long ago life was lovely and normal. Every day was just a day, you made yourself look nice and went out to work, looked after the kids, ran around the house, had spontaneous sex, fitted into your lovely clothes, socialised, had conversations, multi-tasked and were just marvellous. Your skin was dewy and glowing. Your stomach muscles still worked.

Then, without any particular notice or warning, you woke up and found yourself looking at your lovely life from a hazy distance. You looked down and realised you were waist deep in a sea of shit.

It hurt to move but you had to wade through the shit to get dressed and get out of the house. You squeezed your aching joints into clothes that were suddenly and alarmingly too tight.

You had developed a giant fanny tummy – just one mass of bloat from your waist to your flaps - which was straining to burst out of your jeans. Feeling like you had been squeezed into a sausage skin, you plodded through the shit to get to the mirror.

You tried to put make up on but your face had apparently been boiled overnight and resembled a red, bloated old women's face who looked like she had been drinking 3 litres of park bench cider every day for 50 years. She looked a bit like you so you looked again, to be sure, and saw that the woman had whiskers on her chin, a 3-inch wayward eyebrow hair and the beginnings of a fine moustache.

You also had a fine crop of nasal hair.

Plucking the hair made you sneeze.

Sneezing made you piss.

You looked down and realised that, hidden by the sea of shit, your pelvic floor had quite possibly dropped out of your insides and was hanging around somewhere in the region of your knees. And your knees now had thick black hair on the back of them.

Before you could scream 'What the fuck is happening?' you forgot what you were going to say and burst into tears.

Creaking down the stairs in your sausage skin jeans with your alcoholic old lady hairy face you made it through the sea of shit to the kitchen.

Everybody was happy and chirpy and normal.

This pissed you off big time.

Can't they see that you are in trouble?

But, no, scant attention is paid and you realise your suffering is invisible, you are stuck on the horizon of normal life separated by the shit sea, flailing around trying to keep on keeping on.

And so, begins the menopause or peri-menopause. You bloat, you ache, you cry, you rage, you sweat, you forget, you struggle. You grow hair faster than you can pluck it. Your fandango dries up or develops a cycle of UTI's. You piss yourself. You fart anywhere and everywhere as if it is the most normal thing in the world. Fuck it, you tried holding one in a few times and damn near shit yourself so now you let them go loudly and proudly, defying anyone to challenge you by giving them the death glare.

You drive angry, it is impossible to have a nice pootle along in your car and enjoy driving; you are hunched over the wheel in a permanent fury like Dick Dastardly with Tourette's shouting FUCKHEAD! SHITHEAD! WANKER! BOLLOKS! PRICK! ARSE! COCKSUCKER! KNOB! on repeat, even if you are just reversing the car off the drive.

Occasionally the shit sea will send you a life line on its tide – perhaps HRT or magic patches or some medication that makes you feel like you again, and so you inch a bit closer, through the shit to the shore, giving those of us still stuck a thumbs up of encouragement.

More often the shit sea will just push you further away from yourself on a current of hot flushes, anxiety, more weight gain and insomnia. It really helps, at times like this, when some helpful soul reminds you that they have always been a size 8, never had a beard and think they might've had one hot flush for 20 seconds 2 years ago but it could've just been the oven door opening. When this happens, you say FUCK OFF a lot, but mostly in your head because, despite the shit sea, you are still quite a nice, kind person and don't like hurting other people's feelings.

You have no strength or energy to even try to fight your way through the shit so you just bob around in it, waiting for the awfulness to pass. This might take years; it might never fully pass. In despair, you join online groups and find your people. You are not alone in the sea of shit! The more you talk about it, the better you feel until, one day, the shit sea has receded just enough for you to claw your way back to yourself.

You are different, but you have survived. You plop back into your life as if you never left. Energy and motivation return, and you find that you have regained the ability to love yourself. You might always smell a bit of pee, and fart without warning; there will always be a rouge eyebrow hair and your eyesight has gone to shite so you can no longer see your chin bristles, you just absent mindedly run your fingers over them, like reading braille.

You will always need KY Jelly and piss pads. You will never wear hot pants for fear of wispy growler hair escaping from a slackened flap. However, you accept these as battle scars from the war against the menopause, and are just grateful you are not still floundering in the shit sea.

Life returns slowly to something resembling normality. You think about retiring, gardening, bird tables, and baking. You think you are done with all those wild mood swings and nasty language.

Until you get in your car. Like a reflex, your shoulders hunch up ready to fight and your mouth lets fly a wonderful stream of obscenities before you have turned the ignition on.

Yes, you are still fabulous and thank fuck for that.

The Cloud
26th January 2023

Anybody else feeling like they have been living under a cloud recently? A big, dark, fucked off thundercloud that follows you around everywhere? It weighs your shoulders down and makes you slump.

It makes you snarl and snap at everyone.

It makes everything get right on your tits.

It makes you not want to do any personal grooming. Let it go feral. Why should you spend your best years shearing that fur ball every other day? If he can't handle hacking his way in to get a treat then too bad.

You feel irritated and irked and proper pissed off.

There is a core of rage simmering away inside and it takes all your effort to keep the lid on it. Otherwise, you will blow and not in the way your husband likes on his birthday.

I don't know if I am feeling like this because it is still January, because I am on a diet, because of the menopause or just because I am a moody cow who has moods.

But I feel proper narky.

I quite like it.

But nobody else does, so, in order to get rid of the cranky cloud, I decided to go to Aqua fat last night.

Due to the lack of personal grooming, I carefully spent time painstakingly tucking my stragglers inside my costume.

To maintain my ladylike image, I was sure to do this in the toilets. I was in there for 3 hours.

I haven't been to Aqua fat for ages and, although it was always good fun it used to be quite a tame work out. The hot tub posse would sit there, boiling like crabs in a pot, hoping to catch a glimpse of boob as we merrily did our star jumps. One wrinkled bloke even reclined himself on a sun lounger every week, all the better to get a front row view. 30 women jumping about and giving him the death glare while smiling like synchronised swimmers to show our instructor we were enjoying the class was quite a sight to behold.

However, I strolled in last night to find a new instructor. Very petite and pretty with a lovely way about her, even though she was half the age and half the size of the average class attendee I couldn't help liking her at once.

Alas, lurking underneath this charming exterior was a cross between Windsor Davies and Mr Motivator. Literally seconds into the class, a tidal wave of water had sloshed over the side of the pool as ladies of a certain age and size ran, boxed, danced, jumped, squatted, lunged and twisted, all of us wondering what the fuck was happening.

I did things I didn't even know I could do.

There was no time to worry about a boob escaping and even sun lounger man, fearful of a tsunami, had taken flight.

Our instructor was high on power, urging us on doing all the moves poolside with an endless supply of energy. She reminded me of my mad cocker spaniel puppy, turning round in circles, jumping, running backwards and forwards, everywhere all at once, madly enthusiastic.

There was no stopping her.

My carefully tucked in pubes escaped and nearly ensnared my neighbour, like jellyfish tentacles. The drag weighed me down a bit so I had to work twice as hard.

But it was a fabulous class, the best I have been to, and the cranky cloud lifted up and away a little bit.

I might even do some growler landscaping in time for next week. Either that or put it in a French braid.

Self Help
5th February 2023

I am quite often asked on this page is such and such is a symptom of menopause. So, I have decided to complete a list of things that, as far as I am aware, have only decided to shit on me since the menopause started.

Brain fog. This covers a wide ranging array of issues. Purse in the fridge? Can't remember something? Answering the remote control? Inability to focus? Forgot what you were saying half way through saying it? Welcome to Brain Fog. It is shit, nothing good to see here.

Helpful tip: try to forget that you have brain fog.

Weight gain. It is not your imagination; middle aged spread is a thing. Just as you feel your most unattractive and undesirable mother nature makes you fat. You can exercise 20 hours a day or have it all sucked out and placed into your lips. Or you can say fuck it and eat chips.

Helpful tip: Make new friends who are bigger than you.

Sex drive: Your hormones are up and down like a whore's drawers. You will have zero interest for weeks, even months. You feel dried up and past your sell by date. And then, suddenly at 20 past 3 on a Wednesday, and for no reason at all, you will be hornier than a sailor on shore leave. Alas, by the time you have personal groomed and blown the dust of the KY Jelly, the urge will have flown.

Helpful tip: Get the other half to wear a blindfold and oven gloves – he will neither see nor feel the great growler growth.

Pubic hair: Grey and wiry. You might have spent your adult years cultivating a lovely lush bush, or, every time a pube so much as reared its head, you may have gone into a frenzy of waxing, shaving, hair removing to have a biff like a billiard ball. It is all for nothing. One day you will have a wire wool saggy granny fanny. Sorry.

Helpful tip: get fat so you can't see your fanny and don't look at anything below the waist in the mirror.

Farting. I don't know if there is a medical reason for why your arsehole goes as slack as a windsock on a sunny day, but there will come a time when you will not be able to hold in even the smallest, most humble of farts. You will fart getting up. You will fart walking around. If you try to let out a sneaky one in a crowded room it will develop into a 30 second rip roarer.

Helpful tip: Say PARDON YOU! very loudly to the person next to you and wave your hand frantically in their direction.

Incontinence. Like your arsehole, your pelvic floor will slacken with age until it is neither use nor ornament. It might make a half arsed effort to hold in some pee when you sneeze, only to release a gallon of it should you have the audacity to sneeze again. Remember the glory days when you used to say 'Bless me' when you sneezed? Now you say 'For Fucks Sake' and dash as fast as you can, crab like, to the nearest loo to mop up.

Helpful tip: Try piss pads and avoiding people who say their pelvic floor is the same as it was at 16.

Skin. Perhaps you used to be the happy owner of a glowing and dewy complexion? Now you are wearing a red, broken veined, saggy jawed, permanent resting bitch face, wrinkled Halloween mask. Except you can't take the fecking thing off. Helpful tip: Try Aldi caviar anti-wrinkle cream and learn to apply make up in the dark so you don't have to see the naked face in the mirror.

Aching. Hips, knees, back, feet. It is horrible feeling like a 90-year-old when you are supposed to be in the prime of your life. Every time you get out of bed you question whether or not you need a hip/knee replacement or both. It is not possible to move without making a deep, guttural groaning sound.

Helpful tip: Stay in bed or take up lovely yoga.

Itching. I don't know why this happens, but, at times, it does feel like you have fleas and head lice crawling all over you with the sole intention of driving you bonkers.

Helpful tip: Live in a swimming pool, try an antihistamine, or use Sudocrem and shampoo for an itchy scalp.

Insomnia. Just awful, and is always worse when you are bone achingly tired. Made worse by your partner immediately falling asleep and rubbing your face in it by snoring like a 747 on take-off.

Helpful tip: Shove that snoring bastard into another room to sleep, try a herbal sleep remedy, remind yourself it won't last forever.

Anxiety. Horrendous. How can you go from a happy go lucky, confident, capable woman to a hunched over crone consumed with worry about everything? It is one of the cruellest symptoms of menopause and obviously no help at all with insomnia.

Helpful tip - And this is perhaps the only non-tongue in cheek suggestion: Do not watch the news or read a newspaper, try anti-anxiety meds, yoga, massages and look into alternative healing like crystals, meditation etc.

Facial hair. At some point, without warning you will develop a moustache, nasal hair and a nice bit of a chin stubble including thistle bristles – spiky, stubborn and with the ability to rapidly multiply the more you pluck them out. At around the same time, a wire wool pubic hair will migrate from your granny fanny and attach itself to your left eyebrow. It will be white, three inches long, have the texture of a Brillo pad and will remain hidden until you need to have a very important conversation with somebody. Then it will uncoil and blow gently in the breeze.

Helpful tip: wear a scarf and always carry tweezers.

Mood swings. Angry, fuming, crying, happy, miserable, depressed, happy, laughing, pissed off, upset, manic, joyful. All in the space of 2 minutes. It is not your fault, you and your hormones are riding a rollercoaster you didn't ask to get on and cannot get off.

Helpful tip: really, there is only Gin or the drink of your choice to turn to, plus your girlfriends who will love you regardless.

Not giving a shit. Hurrah! At last, something to be grateful for. That and my tastebuds falling in love with Gin at around the age of 45. You suddenly have the power to make big life decisions without fearing the consequences. Get rid of that toxic acquaintance, tell the boss to stick it, put yourself first, follow your dreams.

Helpful tip: say Fuck off a lot, and try Fever tree slimline tonic with your gin.

A Little Old Man
9th February 2023

So, I was trying to get a bit spicy in the bedroom and found a pair of fishnet tights I didn't know I had.

I hadn't shaved my legs and couldn't be bothered to go through the whole rigmarole; therefore tights presented the perfect solution.

Feeling like a devil, I got handy with the scissors and made the fishnets crotchless. Then snipped away a bit more so my bum could hang out.

I tried them on.

I felt sexy and ready to rumble.

But then, alas, alas, I broke every rule in the book and looked in the mirror to see what the hairy Mary looked like in her new, DIY crotch free home. She felt sexy, naughty, liberated and unrestrained. Surely, she would look glorious?

Holy mother.

Fuck a doodle do.

I instantly thought of a squashed, grumpy, wrinkled and bearded old man peering angrily through his net curtains.

Lights and tights off it was then.

A middle age woman woke up one day

Her memory was shit and her pubes were grey

One minute she was happy the next so sad

She was fecking boiling and her temper was bad

There were aches in her hip and pains in her knee

She lost the ability to hold in her pee

Her perfume was replaced by a vague smell of piss

With her five o'clock shadow she was hard to miss

A nice roll of fat, a tube of lube

And big black hairs around her boob

Celebs are great and try to reassure

All while wearing a UK size 4

Energetic, exercise, perky and strong

I feel I am doing the menopause wrong.

I sit on the sofa with my biscuit stash

Wiping the crumbs out from my moustache

I don't want to skip or spin like a top

I'd only pee and reach for the mop

I'll just sit back and take it all in

Farting and sipping a big glass of gin

Printed in Dunstable, United Kingdom

75185398R00090